*The Psychedelic Anthology* is a seven-part anthology and collection of real-life psychedelic experiences shared from all over the world. This anthology challenges the negative stigma surrounding sacred medicines such as LSD, Ayahuasca, and Mescaline by sharing the very profound and transformative experiences that may occur while under the influence of these substances, many of which have been used as sacraments in religious and spiritual ceremonies for millennia to heal and connect with the divine. Through these incredibly powerful stories, this book series hopes to humanize these medicines and reintroduce their importance to mankind.

## Disclosure

The sole purpose of *The Psychedelic Anthology* is to share people's real-life experiences with different psychedelic substances. In doing so, the creator of this book is not condoning, encouraging, or recommending their use and shall not be held liable or accountable for any loss, injury, or damage allegedly arising from the reading or discussing of this book's content. Furthermore, it is important to understand that the use of the substances mentioned in this book may lead to psychological or physical harm if used irresponsibly or improperly. As a reader, please be aware that the legality of the psychedelic substances discussed herein varies, and in different municipalities the possession, sale, or use of these substances may lead to a fine or imprisonment.

Interior Art by Stuart Holland
www.stuarthollandart.com

Cover Art "Healer" by Heather McLean
www.hbomb.ca

Library of Congress Control Number: 2016955613

To
Change

A special thanks to **Psymposia** and all of the contributors for sharing their experiences.

*Introduction*

*The Experiment at La Chorrera*       7

*The Experiences*

*The Other Side of Yesterday*       37

*The Screaming Abyss*       53

*The Key*       71

*Life is But a Dream*       75

*The Resistance Had to End If I Was to Begin*       83

*Impermanent Immortality*       93

*Transformation Through Death & Rebirth*       99

*Return to the Tree of Knowledge*       105

*Heart Medicine*       109

*It Is What It Is*       115

Show Me the True Nature of the Universe      119

Honoring My Inner Goddess      183

Relaxing With What Is      187

Marinating in the Essential Stew      199

MDMA Therapy for Rape Trauma      207

A Red Marble Sky      217

The New Birth      225

Ditching My Crutches & Scaling Mountains      231

Awakening to the Infinite      235

Unplugging From the Matrix      241

Waves of Love      249

A Night of Beauty and Bliss      253

Into the Source of Death Anxiety      265

*2001: LSD Odyssey*      299

*Depression, Alcoholism, and Ayahuasca*      305

*Cosmic Explosion*      319

*My Rebirth*      325

*Master Plant Dieta*      329

*The Ancient Forest*      349

*Dissolving the Illusion*      359

*The Crystal Towers*      367

*Earth, The Grand Stage*      375

*APPENDIX*

# The
# Psychedelic
# Anthology

## Volume II

# *Introduction*

# THE EXPERIMENT
# AT LA CHORRERA

*The following story consists of excerpts from "The Brotherhood of the Screaming Abyss" by Dennis McKenna about an experience with psychedelics that he shared with his late brother Terence McKenna during their 1971 trip to La Chorrera.*

Mission La Chorrera consisted of a small church with a wooden bell tower, the padre's residence, a police outpost near the dock on the river, and a cluster of buildings that included classrooms and a few other simple structures. The padre, a Capuchin priest by the name of Father José Maria, let us stay temporarily near the mission in a hut on stilts we quickly dubbed the "knoll house." In a few days, the padre told us, the families would depart and there would be numerous empty dwellings to choose from. We had our eyes on another raised hut set off in the forest, but until that opened we were quite happy where we were. The knoll house stood on a rise perhaps two hundred yards away from the mission but still in the pasture, a large area cleared from the forest to accommodate a herd of humped zebu cattle. The riverbank was about one hundred yards from the knoll.

The combination of pastures, cattle, and frequent warm rains had created an ideal habitat for Psilocybe cubensis. These mushrooms are known to be pan-tropical; they occur in both hemispheres, in any place with a warm climate where cattle are raised; in fact, they can be considered symbionts of the cattle, whose dung provides a rich substrate for them. *Psilocybe cubensis*, then classified as *Stropharia cubensis*, are the most widespread and common of the tropical Psilocybin mushrooms. We found them growing everywhere in the pastures around the knoll house and beyond. There were big, beautiful clusters of carpophores sprouting out of nearly every cowpat, quite impossible to ignore. We must have arrived at the peak of the season; earlier in our trip we'd only spotted a few specimens. Needless to say, we were delighted at this unexpected good fortune.

The specimens were succulent and quite delicious, their slight bitterness easy to overlook in light of our scant food supplies. We'd brought rice, beans, and tinned meats, wrongly assuming we'd be able to purchase other foods along the way. We could buy fruit, eggs, and yuca, or manioc root, from the locals, and condensed milk and noodles from the tiny tienda at the mission, but our diet was spare and boring. We found that a few mushrooms added to boiled rice or an omelet provided just the thing to perk up an evening's meal; and the best thing was that the after-dinner entertainment was built in.

We had not yet understood that the mushrooms were the real Secret. We regarded them much too casually as mere recreation. As a result we found it very easy to eat them daily, either as part of the meal or as a mid-afternoon snack, with no immediate adverse effects. They were an excellent complement to the cannabis, which we smoked constantly, along with the occasional hit derived from shavings taken from our fresh supply of *Banisteriopsis caapi,* the vine added to Ayahuasca as a source of MAO-inhibiting compounds. We found that smoking the bark while on mushrooms synergized the closed-eye hallucinations in a most pleasant and intriguing way. We dubbed this serendipitous discovery "vegetable television."

It didn't take too many days of such behavior for events to evolve in some fairly peculiar directions. As anyone with experience will tell you, the mushrooms stimulate conversation, and they give one "funny ideas" that seem to be quite novel, even hilarious. Being constantly on a low dose of mushrooms gave new verbal agility to an already very verbal bunch. Our conversations, full of non sequiturs and amusing puns, flowed freely and more or less remained in this noetic space all the time. It was as if our group of five had been joined by an extremely erudite, clever, and delightful guest who had come for dinner and decided to stay.

The mushrooms encouraged the wildest intellectual fantasies, as if egging us on to ever more outlandish scenarios. We heatedly discussed the parallels between alchemical fluids and crystals and shamanic phlegm. We also explored the role played by sound in evoking these phenomena. Anyone who has smoked DMT can testify that sounds heard inside the head are a prominent part of the experience. Sometimes the sounds are like ripping cellophane, sometimes they are more like electrical sounds, buzzing, popping, and humming noises. Not uncommonly, similar sounds are often heard on high doses of mushrooms. As Terence noted, DMT seems to trigger glossolalia and other forms of spontaneous vocalization. Once the interior sound is perceived, there is an impulse to imitate it with the voice, to sing along with it. The sound doesn't lend itself well to imitation, but if one tries, the voice eventually seems to lock on to the inner buzz, which then pours out of one's mouth in a long, powerful ululation that is quite alarming and unlike any sound one would ordinarily utter. And making the sound is cathartic. It triggers an almost orgasmic ecstasy, and it greatly stimulates the closed-eyelids visual phenomena. There is a precedent for this in the traditions of Ayahuasca shamanism as well. The Icaros, the healing songs sung by Ayahuasqueros, are used to evoke the inner visions and thereby direct the inner journey. There is apparently a tight link between the Icaros and the inner visions, and the manifestation of these fluid psycho-substances.

Our conversations revolved around these heady ideas night after night as we communed with our new companion. And by then we did have a sense of being in the presence of an "other," an entity of some kind that was fully participating in the conversation, though in a nonverbal or perhaps metalinguistic way. We came to think of this other as "the Teacher," though it was unclear whether that meant the mushrooms themselves, or if the mushrooms provided a channel for communicating with some unidentified entity. Whatever it was, the Teacher was full of interesting suggestions about how our investigations should proceed. We began to think pure Logos had taken physical form, that is, manifested itself as a substance composed of mind, of language, of meaning itself, yet all somehow grounded in a biological substrate. We used the term "translinguistic matter" to describe this mysterious substance, and we speculated that somehow it was produced in the peculiar state created by ingesting tryptamines. We figured this matter was Psilocybin or DMT that had been "rotated" through the fourth dimension so that its "trip" was on the outside of the molecule. The same way a piece of sheet music is made up of printed notes on a page.

The notes are an abstract way of denoting sounds of a particular pitch and duration, played in a particular sequence. The sheet music is a representation of the music, in effect a schematic diagram of the music, but not music per se. The music manifests itself when the notes are played in a process unfolding through time – the fourth dimension. The more we kicked around these concepts, the more excited we became.

On our seventh night at La Chorrera, the idea of my body being an instrument became all too real after I'd taken nineteen mushrooms, my largest dose yet. As Terence put it, I suddenly stiffened and "gave forth, for a few seconds, a very machine-like, loud, dry buzz" accompanied by what I felt to be an intense welling of energy. In many ways, this was the moment when the weirdness leapt to another level.

In retrospect, I see how our conceits embodied a paradox of the psychedelic experience. On one level we understood that a molecule doesn't "contain" the trip. Rather, the trip is an interaction between a living organism and a molecule's pharmacological properties. These properties may be inherent to the drug, but the trip itself is not. That explains why a drug manifests differently in different organisms, and even differently in the same organism at different times.

We got that, sort of. But in our delusion, if that's what it was, we also embraced a conflicting view: We believed an intelligent entity resided in the drug, or at least somehow communicated to us through it. Even as we theorized about the 4-D expression of the drug – that the trip could somehow be expressed on its exterior by rotation through the fourth dimension – we were assuming on another level that a being of some sort was directing the trip.

We weren't the first or the last to make that "mistake." After all, this is very close to shamanistic views of the psychedelic experience, in which the drug speaks through a skilled practitioner. Though psychedelics have been widespread for decades, people still have a natural tendency to describe their experiences as though the trip were in the drug: "The LSD gave me wonderful visions," they might say, or "Ayahuasca showed me," or "The mushrooms told me." I'm keenly aware how seductive this assumption is, and how easily I slip into it myself, if only as a figure of speech. And yet as a scientist I must say no: These substances did none of those things. The human mind-brain created these experiences. At La Chorrera, the Psilocybin somehow triggered metabolic processes that caused a part of our brains to be experienced not as part of the self, but as the "other" – a separate, intelligent entity that seemed to be downloading a great many peculiar ideas into our consciousness.

That's the reductionist perspective. Is it true? I honestly can't say, even today. It either is true, or the alternative is true, that there actually are entities in "hyperspace" that can communicate with us via something akin to telepathy when the human brain is affected by large amounts of tryptamine. That's a hypothesis worthy of testing, if such an experiment could ever be devised.

But at La Chorrera, we couldn't be bothered with such nuances. Believing the mushroom, or the Teacher, to be urging us on, we conjured up our theory about what was happening and then resolved to test it. Our "experiment" was not to prove if the Teacher existed. We took that for granted. We wanted to see if what the Teacher was teaching us would really deliver.

I should clarify that by "we" I don't mean our entire party. Life in the shadow of the little mission had taken some interesting turns. Vanessa and Dave had moved out of the knoll house to a hut nearer the river. Meanwhile, on March 2nd, Terence, Ev, and I had moved farther away, down the trail to the forest hut, which by then had opened. The split, while friendly, suggested a philosophic divide. Some of us wanted to run with the ideas we were entertaining, and some did not. I should add that the ideas "we" were entertaining were largely mine. Dave and Vanessa were clinging to the reductionist view for all they were worth; the weirdness around us could all be explained, they said, in familiar, psychological terms. The rest of us were suiting up for a plunge into another dimension.

We decided our experiment would occur on the evening of March 4th. Terence spent much of March 3rd gathering dried roots and sticks from the area around our new hut for our experiment. On the appointed morning, he used that to build a large fire and boil up some Ayahuasca from the plants he'd brought back from the Witoto village. I had it on the Teacher's authority that the beta-carbolines in Ayahuasca, present as harmine, might be the special seasoning we needed to make the recipe work, a key component in whatever it was we were concocting. Years later, in his account, Terence would question whether his brew had really been strong enough to "provoke an unambiguous intoxication." His theory was that the MAO inhibiting effect of harmine might have potentiated the

Psilocybin we still had in our systems from the large doses of mushrooms we'd already taken. It's worth noting that we hadn't ingested any mushrooms for a couple of days preceding the experiment. Whatever the reason, the abyss had opened, and we were going in.

Whether the ideas that seized us over those days were telepathically transmitted by the mushroom, or by a mantis-like entity on the bridge of a starship in geosynchronous orbit above the Amazon (which we considered), or created within our own minds, I'll never know. I do know that our lively discussions led us to speculate about how the phenomenon might be assessed. I should clarify that. By then, the Teacher had suggested the outlines of an experiment to me.

Or I believed so anyway, in my state of hypermania. Wildly stimulated by the concepts at play, I felt I was downloading explicit instructions from the Teacher, the mushroom, or whatever it was, about our next steps. The goal wasn't simply to test the hypothesis but to fabricate an actual object within the alchemical crucible of my body. This thing would be a fusion of mind and matter created by the fourth-dimensional rotation of the metabolizing Psilocybin and its exteriorization, or "freezing," into a physical object. Such an object would be the ultimate artifact. It would be the philosopher's stone, or the UFO space-time machine, or the resurrection body – all these things being conceptualizations of the same thing. The Teacher was downloading the blueprints for building a hyper-dimensional vehicle out of the 4-D transformation of my own DNA interlaced with the DNA of a mushroom. But not just blueprints alone. I was also getting step-by-step instructions on how to build this transcendental object.

The information that was downloaded to me by the Teacher was a recipe for constructing a hyperdimensional artifact that would bind four dimensions into three and thereby end history. An object made of mushrooms, bark, and my own DNA, welded together using the sound of my voice. The Teacher was blunt: "If you do this procedure, it will happen." Build it, and they will come; more precisely, build it, and you will hold all of space-time in your hands, in the form of the stone. The philosopher's stone – singing to a mushroom while completely ripped on high doses of Psilocybin boosted with harmine from the Ayahuasca – will make manifest the most miraculous object imaginable. Mind and matter will fuse into a hyper-dimensional object that is the ultimate artifact at the end of time, whose very creation brings an end to time, leading humanity to a state in which all places and all times are instantly accessible at the speed of thought. It's crazy stuff. It reads like the ravings of an unhinged mind, and perhaps that's what it was. There's more:

> There comes a time...that time has come. History will end in a few hours. The day itself has ordained the command to humankind: March Fourth. March Forth, humanity, to greet a new dawn, as you slid and swam and crawled and walked down the spiral chains of evolutionary metamorphosis to your final awakening. For this is the day when you will sleep no more: you have been blinded by the black veil of unconsciousness... for for the last time.

Why I and my companions have been selected to understand and trigger the gestalt wave of understanding that will be the hyperspatial zeitgeist is becoming more clear to me each moment, though I know I won't understand our mission fully until the work is complete.

We will be instructed in the use of this knowledge by some infinitely wise, infinitely adept fellow member of the hyperspatial community; of that I feel sure. It will be the taking of the keys to galactarian citizenship. I speculate that we will be the first five human beings to be instructed in its use. Our mission will be to selectively disseminate it to the rest of humanity, but slowly and in such a way as to ease the cultural shock. It is also somehow appropriate that at least some segment of the species has an intimation of the implications and possibilities of this, the last cultural artifact. To many it was given to feel the stirrings of change, but to a few only was complete understanding granted in the final hours before the accomplishment: surely so that the last words ever spoken in language in the final hours of history can be a chronicle of the defeat of the oldest tyrant: Time.

And so now, against all the probabilities of chance and circumstance, my companions and I have been given the peculiar privilege of knowing when history will end. It would be a strange position to find oneself in, if being in that position did not bring with it a full understanding of just what forces brought one there. Fortunately, as the phenomenon is an acceleration of understanding, one gains clearer insight into the forces that have bent space and time, and thought and culture back upon themselves to focus them at this point.

Now I can look back upon my life spread before the scanner of memory and understand all those moments that have foreshadowed this one. It is easy to look beyond personal history to all of the events of history, and discern therein the prefiguration of this last moment. As a phenomenon, it has always existed and will continue, as it is a moving edge of phenomenal understanding that was generated with the first atom and has gathered momentum in a constant acceleration ever since. What we are moving toward in 3 dimensions is the passing of the wave of understanding into the fourth dimension, the realm of the atemporal. As it happens, it will make the transition through one of us. But there will be no change in the cosmic order, or even a blip on the cosmic circuits, for the phenomenon has gathered constant momentum from the beginning, and will flow through and beyond the fourth dimension with the same smoothness it entered, until finally it has moved through all beings and all dimensions. Its job will then be complete, when, in a billion eternities, it has constellated full understanding throughout creation.

There is rich material here for the student of pathology. I'm acutely aware of that as I read those words penned so long ago in an Amazonian hut by a much younger Dennis who was utterly convinced he was about to collapse, or at least transcend, the space-time continuum. The ravings of a madman, I'll grant that. And yet, there is also poetry here, and beauty, and a longing for redemption. What I expressed is not that different from the vision articulated by the most compassionate and beautiful of the world's religions: the Universe will not achieve perfection until all beings have achieved enlightenment. Isn't that what I'm saying? No doubt there is messianic delusion here; indeed. But there is also a deep wish for healing, not only of myself but of the Universe. Our mother had been dead less than six months. I have to believe that much of what happened to us at La Chorrera was linked to that tragic event. So overwhelmed were we by the sense of loss, and of guilt, we were ready to tear space and time apart in order to reverse that cosmic injustice.

On the evening of March 4th, Dave and Vanessa joined us for dinner at the forest retreat, but they wanted no part in our looming adventure. The sudden approach of a violent thunderstorm brought us all outside to stare agog at a massive, flickering cloud; then the wind and rain hit, and Vanessa slipped on the wet ladder as she hurried back into our raised hut, hurting her ankle. After the storm passed and Dave and Vanessa had departed, Terence, Ev, and I completed the experiment's final preparations, as dictated earlier by the Teacher. We knew our success was assured, thanks to the strange signs we were given as the moment neared, from the intense lightning to the apparent breach of physical law, including the eerie steadiness of a tilted candle's flame, our only light. These phenomena (or so we told ourselves) were caused by the shockwave of the continuum-destabilizing events, now just hours ahead, as it rippled back into the past like a kind of temporal echo. We were approaching the singularity. We knew we were going to succeed because, just a few hours ahead, we already had.

By then, we'd taken the Ayahuasca off the fire and set it aside, along with some bark shavings from the Banisteriopsis vine we'd used to make it. We planned to drink a small cup of the brew when we ate the mushrooms and, if necessary, smoke the bark to activate and synergize the Psilocybin. Earlier, we'd gone to the pasture and located a beautiful specimen of *Psilocybe cubensis* and carried it back, intact and metabolizing on its cow-pie substrate. We had also collected several perfect specimens we'd eat to initiate the experiment. On the floor of the hut we drew a circle marked with the four cardinal points, and placed drawings of I Ching hexagrams at each one, to define and purify the sacred space where the work was to occur. Inside the circle, we placed the mushroom we'd chosen as our receiving template, along with the Ayahuasca and the bark shavings. We suspended the chrysalis of a blue morpho butterfly near the circle so the metabolizing tryptamine from that source would be present. Why that of all things? We were attempting a kind of metamorphosis, and so clearly we needed a chrysalis close by. Kneeling together in the circle, each of us drank a small cup of the bitter brew, still slightly warm from its preparation. I munched two mushrooms, and we climbed into our hammocks to wait.

By then we were fully in the grip of the archetypal forces we'd activated. We were no longer in profane time or profane space; we were at the primordial moment, the first (and the last) moment of creation. We had moved ourselves to the center of the cosmos, that singularity point at which, as the Hermetic philosophers put it, "What is here is everywhere; what is not here is nowhere." We were not in control any longer, if we ever had been. We were acting out our roles in an archetypal drama.

Though we were motionless, cocooned in hammocks in a hut in the Amazon, it felt as though we were approaching the edge of an event horizon. We could clearly perceive time dilating as we neared the moment of "hyper-carbolation," our term for the act of sonically triggering the 4-D transformation of the blended Psilocybin and beta-carboline. Time was slowing down, becoming viscous as molasses as we fought against the temporal gale howling down from the future. "A series of discrete energy levels must be broken through in order to bond this thing," I said. "It is part mythology, part psychology, part applied physics. Who knows? We will make three attempts before we break out of the experimental mode.

Who knew, indeed? We were following a script, but no longer a script we'd written. I ate one more mushroom and settled back into my hammock, wrapped in my poncho-like ruana. It didn't take long before the mushroom's energy began coursing through my body. I could hear the internal signal tone getting stronger in my head; it had been easy to evoke, never far from perception for the last several days. I was ready to make the first attempt to charge the mushroom template.

I'll let Terence take it from there:

> Dennis then sat up in his hammock. I put out the candle, and he sounded his first howl of hyper-carbolation. It was mechanical and loud, like a bull roarer, and it ended

with a convulsive spasm that traveled throughout his body and landed him out of his hammock and onto the floor. We lit the candle again only long enough to determine that everyone wanted to continue, and we agreed that Dennis's next attempt should be made from a sitting position on the floor of the hut. This was done. Again a long, whirring yodel ensued, strange and unexpectedly mechanical each time it sounded. I suggested a break before the third attempt, but Dennis was quite agitated and eager to "bring it through," as he put it. We settled in for the third yell, and when it came it was like the others but lasted much longer and became much louder. Like an electric siren wailing over the still, jungle night, it went on and on, and when it finally died away, that too was like the dying away of a siren. Then, in the absolute darkness of our Amazon hut, there was silence, the silence of the transition from one world to another, the silence of the Ginnunga gap, that pivotal, yawning hesitation between one world age and the next of Norse mythology. In that gap came the sound of the cock crowing at the mission. Three times his call came, clear but from afar, seeming to confirm us as actors on a stage, part of a dramatic contrivance. Dennis had said that if the experiment were successful the mushroom would be obliterated. The low temperature phenomena would explode the cellular material and what would be left would be a standing wave, a violet ring of light the size of the mushroom cap. That would be the holding mode of the lens, or the philosopher's stone, or whatever it was. Then someone would take command of it – whose

19

DNA it was, they would be it. It would be as if one had given birth to one's own soul, one's own DNA exteriorized as a kind of living fluid made of language. It would be a mind that could be seen and held in one's hand. Indestructible. It would be a miniature universe, a monad, a part of space and time that magically has all of space and time condensed in it, including one's own mind, a map of the cosmos so real that that it somehow is the cosmos, that was the rabbit he hoped to pull out of his hat that morning.

This didn't happen, of course. Nor did a new universe emerge from the Ginnunga gap, the "mighty gap" or abyss or void from which the universe emerged, according to Norse legend. The mushroom did not explode in a cloud of ice crystals as its DNA radically cooled, leaving a softly glowing, lens-shaped hologram humming a few inches above the floor of the hut. That did not happen because it could not happen; such an event would have violated the laws of physics. That didn't bother us in the least – we were convinced we were about to overturn the constraints of conventional physics. Besides, we'd been getting feedback from the future; we knew that we were going to succeed because we already had! Yet what I had confidently predicted didn't occur. What did? Terence again:

> Dennis leaned toward the still whole mushroom standing in the raised experiment area.
> "Look!"
> As I followed his gaze, he raised his arm and across

the fully expanded cap of the mushroom fell the shadow of his ruana. Clearly, but only for a moment, as the shadow bisected the glowing mushroom cap, I saw not a mature mushroom but a planet, the earth, lustrous and alive, blue and tan and dazzling white.

"It is our world."

Dennis's voice was full of unfathomable emotions.

I could only nod. I did not understand, but I saw it clearly, although my vision was only a thing of the moment. "We have succeeded." Dennis proclaimed.

Succeeded at what? Not what I had predicted. But clearly something had happened. For one thing, I think we'd painted ourselves into a metaphysical corner. What I had predicted would happen, could not happen – but we already knew that something would happen, because it already had! I realize this statement suggests a misunderstanding of the nature of time, because how can something that was still in the future have already happened? Nevertheless, this is what we understood.

After the experiment, Terence was confused. I, on the other hand, thought I had the situation well in hand. As dawn neared, we left Ev in the hut and walked out to the pasture in silence, each lost in our own thoughts. I said something to Terence like, "Don't be alarmed; a lot of archetypal things are going to start happening now." And they did. That might have been the last coherent statement I would utter for the next two weeks.

By then I'd begun to disengage from reality, a condition that progressively worsened throughout the day. The reader may quip that we'd been thoroughly disengaged for quite some time, which might have been true; but even what grip I still had was slipping fast. As we stood in the pasture, Terence staring at me quizzically, I said, "You're wondering if we succeeded?" What unfolded over the next few minutes was an episode of apparent telepathy. I could "hear" in my head what Terence was thinking. I was answering his questions before he articulated them, though with or without telepathy they were easy enough to anticipate. All of them were ways of asking, "What the hell just happened?"

But there was more to it than that. I felt I'd manifested a kind of internalized entity, an intelligence now inside me that had access to a cosmic database. I could hear and speak to this oracular presence. I could ask it questions – and get answers. As I explained to Terence, the oracle could be queried by prefacing the question with the name "Dennis." For instance, "Dennis, what is the name of this plant?" And the oracle would instantly respond with a scientific name. Terence soon learned the oracle could also be addressed as "McKenna." Something very peculiar was going on. Whatever it was, we were both under the thrall of the same delusion.

Shortly thereafter I lost my glasses, or rather, I hurled them into the jungle, along with my clothes, in one of my bouts of ecstasy. My blurred vision for the next few weeks surely playing into my estrangement from reality. When I tried to share our wondrous discovery with the others, they were underwhelmed. Vanessa, our resident skeptic, asked some mathematical questions of the oracle, and it was flummoxed, or it gave answers we couldn't verify. Nevertheless, Terence and I were utterly convinced we had succeeded. We were sure that a wave of gnosis was sweeping the world with the advancing dawn line; people were waking up to find themselves, as Terence put it, "pushing off into a telepathic ocean whose name was that of its discoverer: Dennis McKenna."

The events at La Chorrera entered a new phase on our walk that morning in the pasture as we tried to sort out what had happened the night before. My story began with a tremendous journey outward. To the extent that there existed a precedent for what happened to me, I relate it to my DMT trip in Boulder months earlier when I felt my mind had been blown literally to the edges of the Universe. Standing on the lawn that autumn night, I became one with everything; the boundaries of my self were those of the Universe. And so it was as I progressively disengaged from reality over the first day after our experiment at La Chorrera. Once again I was smeared across the totality of space and time. Was I reliving that earlier experience, or having one like it? The question makes no sense. There is only one experience like that, and it is always the same one; it takes place in a moment that is all moments, and a place that is all places.

At any rate, I was back in that place, at that moment. And my reintegration started there as well. I began to "collapse," or perhaps "recondense" is a better term, on what seemed roughly to be a twenty-four-hour cycle; and with each cycle I got that much closer to reintegrating my psychic structure. By the second day I had shrunk to the size of the galactic mega-cluster, and by the third day to that of the local galactic cluster. I continued to condense at that rate down to the size of the galaxy, the solar system, the earth and all its life, the hominid species alone, my ancestral line, and then my family. The final distinction was between my brother and myself. Throughout this ordeal, I hadn't been sure if we were separate entities or not. Once we had separated and I was "myself" again, it wasn't the old self I had left. Like an ancient mariner returning home after a voyage of many years, I was changed forever. I was still resonating with the memories of those experiences, not fully reintegrated by a long shot, but I was grateful to be back in a body, back in a reality that conformed to my expectations – more or less, and most of the time.

But that took a couple of weeks. While I was lost on my shamanic journey, spiraling in closer and closer, Terence was engaged in his own reintegration, in a way that was complementary to mine. I was cruising through multiple spatial dimensions, whereas Terence was anchored in time; he was, in fact, the beacon I was following home. As we understood it, at the moment of hyper-carbolation in our hut on March 4th, we momentarily became one; then we split apart again, in a way that was analogous to the separation of a positive photographic plate from its negative image. We became temporal mirror images of each other. One of us, Terence, was moving forward in time, while I was moving backward in time, from the future. When both of us reached the point where past and future met, we would become fully ourselves again, except that by then we'd have fully integrated the experience of the other. To our companions, what was going on must have presented itself as a classic example of folie à deux, a delusion or psychosis shared by my brother and me. None of us had the vocabulary to describe it at the time; it was only years later that we learned that such phenomena are well documented in the psychiatric literature. What happened to us was certainly a shared altered state, but to reduce it to a mere instance of shared psychosis doesn't really do it justice. I say that even as I know I may still be expressing a compulsion to treat it as something other than that, something more.

But as far as Vanessa and Dave were concerned, the lens of psychiatric illness was the one they reflexively adopted to explain our strange behavior. Because we were acting crazy, we were crazy; and the best solution, as they saw it, was to get us out of that jungle backwater as quickly as possible and into the nearest psychiatric facility. Considering where we were, that option was problematic. I'm grateful that circumstances did not permit it, but I am equally grateful to Terence for resisting the pressure to leave La Chorrera. He insisted that whatever was happening to us be allowed to unfold in its own time and on its own terms. It was clear to him, at least, that I was slowly getting better, and that there was no need for intervention beyond making sure that I didn't wander off or hurt myself. Against her better judgment, perhaps, Vanessa accepted Terence's argument and agreed to a course of watchful waiting. Had my return been interrupted, I doubt that I would have ever "recovered" completely (if that's even the appropriate word). Under the classic model of shamanic initiation, I'd been torn asunder, but I was able to stitch myself back together. There is no telling how things might have gone had the process been aborted.

Over the next few days, we came to assume our alchemical quest had basically succeeded, but that some of our assumptions had been incorrect. The stone we sought to construct, the transcendental object, the lens, had not materialized in a flash. Would that it had! That would have settled the matter. Instead, our success apparently presented itself as a gift for telepathy and access to a vast database not unlike the Akashic Records, the mystical library of all human and cosmic knowledge spoken of by the Theosophists. True, our efforts to validate that knowledge had been problematic, but our connection seemed intact. Our shared line to the Teacher was still open, and we were kept informed, in real time, of what was going down.

We likened this at the time to "how the boar ate the cabbage," our grandfather's phrase for any account that could be trusted as authentic. The Teacher was quite ready to lay down how the boar ate the cabbage. It also insisted we'd gotten everything right, but our timeframe was off. The stone had been created; but because it was by its very nature atemporal, it was tricky to predict just when it would manifest. Part of our task became trying to nail down that moment of "concrescence," that moment when the "ampersand" as we called it then, or the "eschaton" as we dubbed it later – in any case, the last event – would arrive.

Indeed, Terence's effort to predict when and where the stone would appear marked the start of his obsessive ruminations on the nature of time, and the clues to that riddle he believed he'd glimpsed in the I Ching. In his account, Terence remembers the period of my "shamanic ramble" as the most intense time he'd ever gone through. For the next nine days he "neither slept nor needed sleep." He scanned the environment constantly, hoping to catch the stone in the act of concrescence. Willing himself into a state of hyper-vigilance, he also watched me constantly – probably a good thing because I had a tendency to wander away from the hut.

Every day we'd go to the pasture, where Terence would demand that I produce the stone; I couldn't do that, of course, but I predicted it was getting closer and closer. He claims that one reason he made this daily demand of me was to keep me focused on condensing myself as well, which is probably true. I now realize his intense preoccupation with time was as much an integrative process for him as my cosmic homecoming was for me. Both were desperate attempts to get reoriented over the next two weeks; both were more or less successful. This process continued well beyond our departure from La Chorrera; indeed, in some respects, for me it is still ongoing.

On one occasion, I connected with a kind of cosmic telephone exchange that enabled me to ring up anybody I wanted, alive or dead, anywhere in time. One of them was my dead mother, who I reached while she was listening to a radio broadcast of the World Series in 1953. She didn't believe it was me on the line because my nearly three year old self was sleeping in the crib beside her! Other such events seemed to penetrate into the "real world," though at the time that notion seemed very loose indeed. We were living in a situation where the mind was creating reality, or at least modulating reality at a time when it seemed bizarrely susceptible to the force of our imaginations. None of this surprised us; that's what happens when you seize control of the machinery that generates reality. Reality becomes whatever you want it to be.

What we wanted, it seemed, were unexpected electrical phenomena and rainbows without rain, among other quirks of nature. While Terence and I were immersed in our folie à deux, our shared reality, or whatever it was, our companions were puzzled, if not alarmed. Terence and I were communicating telepathically. What was going on was certainly strange, but we understood each other, or so we believed, and these events made sense to us.

The following excerpt is from "A Preliminary Report on an Experiment at La Chorrera," a previously unpublished account we collaborated on, with Terence narrating:

> Dennis evinced enormous mental powers and irritability during the six days following the twenty-eighth; during this time period my own psychology was marked by prolonged states of deep active imagination and "delusions of grandeur." In the early morning hours of March 5th, shortly after the completion of the macroexperiment, the development of both our symptoms took a quantum jump upward. In the space of hardly more than an hour, my brother entered a progressively more detached and cosmic state of essential schizophrenia; this development, coupled with his assurances that this was the proof of the measure of our success, was causing in me a growing certitude that

we had succeeded and that this success meant nothing less than the cessation of all natural limitations in the very near future.

For the next thirty-seven days, especially the next fourteen days, my brother's ideation consisted, among other themes but as a dominant theme, of the idea of a shamanic journey of return, from the ends of space and time, to the earth, with the collected energy configuration of everything condensed into a kind of lens or saucer, a true lapis philosophorum. He projected, and I, experiencing an intense state of reactive paranoid schizophrenia, accepted, the role of God, or father, big brother, or Christ, or, and especially, moral judgment. He in turn manifested an understanding of the principles and methods of science and information control that was truly miraculous. He saw himself at times as a giant computer in a starship making a long journey home under the control of his brother, garbed in the dual role of the cosmic shaman and the Adamic Christ.

From the sixth until the twentieth, neither of us slept, and Dennis raved continuously, in telepathic rapport with anyone he wished, in command of enormous technical erudition and of a strange and rapidly evolving hyperspatial cosmogony. He visualized, following a Manichean perception, the solar system as a huge light pump wherein the light of souls was pumped from planet to planet until it finally leaves the solar system altogether and is transmitted to the home lens at the galactic center. Some of his discoveries included that the Saturnian moon Titan is composed of hashish which resonates with the living mycelium of Psilocybin culture, that tryptamine fish swim in the harmine seas of Neptune, and, most important, that Jupiter is the reflected image of Earth in hyperspace, is teeming with bizarre life forms, and is somehow an essential key to unraveling the racial fate. Late twentieth century history was seen by Dennis as a frantic effort to build an object which he called "the lens" to allow life to escape to Jupiter on the heels of an impending geomagnetic reversal.

Slowly, as the shamanic voyager neared his home, his place in space, his stitch in time, the symptoms faded in each of us. However, the continuing process of understanding triggered by our experiment did not cease. Rather, it continued to exponentially accelerate with the passage of each twenty-four-hour cycle, leading us out of the fantastic ideation of the early days following the experiment.

During that period just after our experiment, I spent most of my time wandering in my own private world; my contact with anyone else's was tangential and occasional. That's a crucial difference between what Terence thought I was experiencing and what I really was experiencing. My thoughts and deeds in what I understood to be hyperspace were far more real to me than external events, even the anomalous ones I participated in and may have caused. But however real those internal processes seemed, they are hard to reconstruct, partly because they lack sequential structure, a chronology that would lend my fragmented memories some coherence. That Terence retained a chronological sense of the interlude in question is another clue to our different experiences. There were times when my rants or just my wild gaze, absent my glasses, brought him "brief stabs of despair," he writes. He'd been reminded again how far away was the place from which I had to return. Nevertheless, he clung to his position that I was steadily getting better and just needed some time.

# The
# Experiences

# THE OTHER SIDE
# OF YESTERDAY

## Ayahuasca

*First Kill*

I was on duty the night Alex decided to commit suicide in the communal showers.

I had reluctantly graduated from the Combat Medics course and returned to my unit for the eighteen months of training left to qualify as "combat ready" and become a fighting member of the Israel Defense Forces.

It was 5 a.m. and I was four hours into my shift. The desert was mute and so was I, as I scanned the rocks and lonely bushes beneath the old lookout tower. The silence was abruptly disturbed by a loud metallic noise. My heart skipped a beat, and my whole body tensed up. I peered into my night vision goggles and listened to the radio.

Being a new recruit, I didn't have the courage to abandon my position without a "good reason," so I decided to call in the disturbance and waited. Seconds after that, I heard the first cries for help; a young soldier screaming for a doctor. The entire base came to life. I ran down the tower as fast as I could towards the commotion. More and more dazed soldiers appeared from their old and shabby brown tents.

I set foot on the scene moments after the arrival of the

on-call doctor. Wearing thick glasses and panting heavily, he seemed to be in control and well accustomed to these situations, perhaps.

The shower walls were smeared with dark red blood. In the middle of the room, the body of a young man laid trembling on the cold white floor. Alex had shot himself just underneath his chin, aiming upwards, with his personal M16 assault rifle.

Half of his face was blown to bits, but somehow he was still breathing. I gasped. I breathed through the nausea and tried to regain my equilibrium. I saw the doctor kneeling beside him. My training kicked in. We proceeded to perform a cricothyrotomy in order to establish a patent airway and administered fluids to raise his heart rate. The doctor shouted out orders; I obeyed. We called in a helicopter for emergency medical evacuation in hopes to get Alex to the nearest civilian hospital in time. He needed to be in an operating room.

Outside I could hear Alex's best friend from home shouting. I heard others trying to prevent him from entering the room. I noticed the smell of the detergents used to clean the showers earlier that evening and the smell of the alcohol we were using to sterilize our medical instruments, but most of all I smelled the blood.

The trauma was too severe and Alex took his last breath. I called off the helicopter. The doctor covered Alex's face with a cloth.

Alex died moments before sunrise. The last thing he must have heard was the hysterical cries of his fellow young recruits who were kept away from the barracks and at a safe distance by the senior staff.

*Everything seemed dreamlike.*

I sat next to his body for a moment, for as long as I could, before my legs decided to take me as far as possible from what now felt like a crime scene that lacked a clear perpetrator, one without a criminal, the scene of a crime where everybody took it upon themselves to become the victim. I could not stand to prepare his body for extraction and went on to wander around the base before realizing that I had abandoned my guard duty.

Frantically, I rushed back to man my post. I was in complete shock. All I could think about was whether or not my commanders knew that I had forsaken my guard duty. Was I in trouble? Was I going to be punished? I climbed up the guard tower and stared into the orange sky, with the Sun slowly rising over the hills of the Negev, Israel's most spectacular landscape.

I did not notice the Commanding Officer approaching my position, as he made his morning rounds. In light of the incident, he stopped to inquire about my wellbeing. He took one look at my pale white face and told me to return to my tent.

There I sat for hours, on the verge of tears, not speaking and not making eye contact with anyone. I sat while Alex was taken to the hospital to be prepared for burial. I sat while the commanding officers undertook the task of damage control. This could be a disastrous blow to the morale of the young recruits in training. I sat as military officials paid a visit to Alex's mother, informing her that her son took his own life. I sat as the army censorship swept the incident under the rug – soldier suicide, for the people's army, is bad press.

Catatonic, I watched the base return to its business-as-usual schedule. Tasks were given, rifles were polished, and breakfast was served.

With my eyes blurry and body weak, I felt a hand on my shoulder. It was my staff sergeant who also happened to be a trained army medic. Staff sergeants are traditionally the toughest members of the unit. They are feared and respected, more so than the officers. I prepared myself for a good old-fashioned army shake up, but he, in a moment of sensitivity and insight, sat beside me and said, "You'll be okay. It's just the beginning. You'll get used to it." I tried to focus my eyes on one point on the ground as he said in a tone-dead voice, "I'm sorry, but this will not be the last person who you will not be able to save, it's just…" He trailed off.

I closed my eyes and nodded. I tried to speak but my throat was too tight. He patted me on the back to motion me to rejoin the squad, which I did. I kept checking up on any news reports regarding Alex's death – there were none to be found. Perhaps it was all just a dream.

## PTSD

It was a Friday winter night several months after the war in Lebanon, and I was once again a civilian. I was, according to the doctors, making my first steps towards what could be described as "feeling normal again."

After the traditional Shabbat prayers and meal, my family turned in for the night. I hugged my mother and wished her goodnight. I was supposed to go out and meet up with some friends for a drink – not the easiest feat for a person who just, a few months earlier, while still in active service, was diagnosed with post-traumatic stress disorder, a common and well-known mental health condition amongst servicemen and women.

The house was quiet with only a few lights left on downstairs. I showered and got dressed. I was just about to leave, shuffling the car keys in my hands, when I inadvertently glimpsed into the mirror. I was startled to find that standing behind me, as reflected in the mirror, was a fully armed and battle-ready Palestinian combatant holding a knife.

I froze. My heart was racing and my palms were sweating. I felt that old and familiar knot forming swiftly in my stomach, anticipating the worst. I was finding it very hard to breathe.

I turned around quickly, completely prepared for what I thought was to be a hand-to-hand combat situation. If I could just deliver a quick disabling blow to his throat or groin I could get to the kitchen in time to draw out a knife and come out of this life-threatening situation victorious.

With my back to the mirror, I quickly realized that no one else was present in the room. I scanned the living room and listened for any strange noises. I crouched and looked under the dining room table and the sofa; the house was empty. But it was not. I know this, with certainty. I saw him. He looked at me. I could smell him. He was preparing to make his move.

I was trying desperately to catch my breath, but then my training took over. I got underneath the dining room table and spent a few minutes surveying the "perimeter," as if I was in a military operation in the West Bank.

The house I grew up in, where my friends and I celebrated birthdays, where I shared my first kiss and played the guitar for hours on end, transformed itself into a battle zone, and we were all in great danger.

I gradually became aware of a dual reality. It was as if half of my brain was processing and reacting to a situation the other half knew was not actually real. This must be what insanity feels like. I tried to focus on things that seemed to be real – family photos, my wristwatch. I tried to breathe. I reminded myself of other occasions where the enemy was not there, where I did not need to hide, where I did not need to fight.

An eternity later, my heart rate and breathing stabilized and I regained control of myself. I calmed down and drank some water to relieve the pain in my throat and smile. Embarrassed. Confused. Alone. I spent the next few days indoors, at home, within walls I tried so very much to trust.

*Healing*

I was lying on the ground. The smell of the fresh, moist soil was comforting and relaxing. Earth. Planet Earth. I was here. I took a deep breath; my lungs filled with sweet cool tropical air. My eyes were closed, but I was absolutely engrossed in the most jaw dropping and somewhat debilitating display of creation. It was as visual as it was emotional; every beam of light was a memory, every geometric shape a trauma, every neon-lit passage a feeling.

Frail and weak, my arms had never been heavier. I almost

couldn't feel them. I wanted to cry but I couldn't. I was intoxicated, I reminded myself and took a deep breath. With my eyes closed, I seemed to close them again and again and then… all seemed to disappear.

With the gracious guidance of the Ayahuasca, on numerous occasions, I have experienced myself leaving my body behind, ascending and transcending, the space-time paradigm of our ordinary state of consciousness. But this experience, this journey, was different… very different.

All I ever wanted in this life, since my experiences in the army and probably before that, was to break free from these mortal shackles of human existence. To break free from the pain, the suffering, and the unbearable anguish, to release myself from the irreconcilable crimes, actions, and deeds we as a species, I as a soldier, have been subjected to and are still committing against each other.

All I wished for was to disappear, become the mythical and the mystical. I hoped to touch the faces of the gods, live amongst the magic, and transform into the mysterious and the divine. Those entities who do not feel, who are not part of the sorrow of man.

All this pain. All this confusion. All this death. I did not want to walk the same path, on the same ground, of those lowly evolved human creatures. I did not want to recognize myself in them. I refused and resisted the very thought of being associated with anything human-especially not with myself.

And so that night I was granted that wish. I received what I was hoping and praying for.

Volume II

My eyes closed. I lost all sense of my body. I found it hard to breathe, the sickening nauseating sensation traveling up and down my spine, in and out of my digestive system and toward my head. It was as painful as it was painless, at times almost enjoyable. I purged. I vomited. I cried. I fainted. I was not alone. There were people there. I could sense them. In and out of this spiraling whirlpool I went. I managed to raise myself to a hammock and was brought water. Everything seemed to be collapsing.

All I wanted to do was to be here, in the ordinary reality. Hear the sounds of the music and the jungle, feel the warmth of the crackling wild bonfire and lay my head down to rest.

All I wanted, all my desire, all my wish was to just be. To be exactly what I am. A human being. An entity of sin and prejudice, fear and loathing, doubt and confusion, destruction and deceit – but also, and more importantly, a pure life form, a sophisticated and grand form of biological life capable of feeling and understanding, a true miracle of nature, a meticulously designed comprehension, full of love, light, empathy, and compassion. A being both dedicated and subjugated to creation, expansion, evolution, and consciousness.

All I wanted was to be there. In my heart. With every living being, soul, spirit, and entity on the face of this planet.

I saw my parents, my sister, and my extended family. I saw myself in the eyes of my mother before I was born. I saw my father in the eyes of his father before he was born, the human family tree and timeline; it was inspiring and vast.

I heard the natives of this land and the indigenous people

in the Middle East, Eurasia, and Africa. I listened to their stories, our stories, my story, without having to hear a word. All that has ever been said has been said in silence.

I felt the tectonic plates in motion, I sensed the plants and flowers blossoming, I heard the roar of the planet Earth, inaudibly directed at us. I was to die. At that moment. My body couldn't take it anymore, it couldn't sustain itself any longer, and it wasn't designed to endure this type of journey. I surrender. I am yours. I am mine. I. Am.

*It all went quiet. Silence. Calm. Gentle.*

The storm had passed. I came back. I came back for more of this human experience. More of everything, more of the misunderstanding and the violence, more of the selfishness and the power struggles, more of the wars and the death – but also, I came back for more of the tenderness, the compassion, and the empathy.

I came back for more Love. I came back for more Life. I exist. And despite all that I have been part of and all that I have seen, I am here, and I am grateful.

I fell in love with my family and friends, tormentors and enemies that night. I fell in love with that piece of land, what people now call the Middle East. I fell in love with the religious fanatics, the Muslims and the Jews as one. I fell in love with the Israeli Military, the Palestinian Militias and the Hezbollah. I fell in love with the crippling corruption and the ongoing ruthless and global financial embezzlement. I fell in love with the broken political parties, the generals, and the profiteers and merchants of war and violence. I fell in love with the sickness, the confusion, and the gripping and seductive fear.

I fell in love with death, as I fell in love with life, as I fell in love with myself.

*Integration*

The Ayahuasca experience is, for many individuals, a daunting experience. But it is also one that could be of great benefit for those who are deeply suffering. The potential is the most important aspect of it, one that is active long before the person actually consumes the substance, or before the person truly understands its botanical origins, its anthropological significance, or natural qualities.

It is the very choice of taking responsibility for your own healing, your own life, for your own state of awareness and being. That in itself is already a gigantic positive step. Perhaps this is where change is born – when you are willing and prepared to work for your sanity, that is when you can start shapeshifting your suffering, and thus reimagining your destiny.

Based on my personal experience dealing with the emotional carnage caused by war and human violence, I believe that the primary, non-neurological aspect of combat-related trauma (and thus the psychological suffering associated with it) has to do with the toxic and debilitating emotional relationship that is formed between the person and the experience of death during those detrimental life events.

The presence of severe levels of violence forces both the physical and psychological experience of death into an extremely narrow paradigm, a limited sphere where every element of the experience is tainted and influenced by the overwhelmingly hostile audio-visual and emotional stimulation present during the traumatic event.

Death, as a psychological, biological, and metaphysical phenomenon, becomes a synonym for destruction, the total annihilation of life, and an occurrence where pain and anxiety are always the predominant features. The ending of physical life can indeed be perceived as a natural and peaceful event, one that is part of the non-threatening aspects of our natural human existence. However, when it is experienced, once or during a prolonged period of time, as a malicious and premeditated act, a calculated and deliberate activity that involves the use of extreme force to dominate and control the "other," it is only natural to expect a multitude of negative emotional and cognitive responses and attitudes towards the phenomenon.

Soldiers, especially those suffering from psychological trauma as a result of experiences endured during their military service, are individuals that ultimately are yearning to be understood; individuals that are longing, on an almost cellular level, to be validated and approved, exonerated and forgiven, ironically and paradoxically, by those who are unfortunately incapable of doing so – the civilian population and, at times, their brothers and sisters in arms, who have had significantly less disruptive emotional responses to the same external events.

My encounters with the Amazonian plant and my experiences with other serotonergic psychedelics revealed to me that I was not able to understand and integrate the experiences and concepts of war, death, and life with my mind alone. I realized that in order to move forward toward true peace and reconciliation, with both myself and all that surrounds me, I will have to learn to use perhaps the most simple and disregarded instrument we have at our disposal – the human heart.

Time after time during my work with the sacred plants and synthetic substances, this realization, at times nauseating and at others blissful, descended upon me with unrelenting force and uncanny persistence. It does so still.

It was clear that my heart had become a muscle that I had forgotten how to use.

Made redundant by the circumstances of my external and internal reality, this heart was closed, on lock down. But, curiously, at the same time of understanding these aspects regarding my own way of being, unconsciously and almost unwillingly, my heart began to open. It imploded, with grace and humility. It blossomed and came to life.

These revelations and understandings, accompanied by many other deep insights and precious moments of epiphany, were fundamental to my process of healing and self-discovery. I was able to heal my relationship with death, and that in turn allowed me to heal my relationship with life.

I have come to acknowledge the tremendous positive psychological properties and qualities of both natural and synthetic psychoactive substances such as the Amazonian Ayahuasca, the Mexican Peyote, the African Iboga, and the Psilocybin mushroom among other plants.

I feel that these precious plants and other healing substances, such as LSD and MDMA, possess a potential so vast, so absolutely critically important for the evolution of human consciousness, for the understanding of the very notion of biological life, that it is nothing less than a perfect Aristotelian tragedy that we, as developed and modern societies, criminalize and prohibit their use.

I feel that the predominant psychological and spiritual experience produced by these wonderfully mysterious substances is one of unity – with oneself, the other, and the environment. It is an inclusive experience. They most often promote and inspire an interdependent state of being that is harmonious and peaceful, positive and trusting, innocent and loving.

When one is for all, all is for one.

In contrast to the aforementioned, it seems noteworthy to mention that in many modern nations, the systematic breakdown of the utopian, social society, welfare state has led to the now entrenched absence of the very concept of community (in this context, a security net) from the daily lives and collective psyche of their citizens. Countless individuals find themselves in a mode of being that is most commonly associated with economic segregation and vulnerability, lacking a socially acceptable personal identity and living in a state of physical insecurity and fear of social exclusion.

The post-industrial era is dangerously disconnected from the most natural and fundamental physical and spiritual needs of this planet and its inhabitants, and therefore there is a real and urgent need to reassess and reevaluate our current paradigms of personal, social, and national existence. Whether the therapeutic or ceremonial ingestion and consumption of these substances takes place in the Amazon rainforest, the hills of Samaria, or in a studio apartment overlooking the Hudson River, they are always celebrated within a group of people. A community that comes together, occasionally or regularly, knowingly or unknowingly, to practice a way of being that is more aware, more understanding, and most importantly, more compassionate. They come together to share a peak experience, a mystical one that has a tremendous amount of therapeutic value. They come together, if only for a few moments, in a man-made world where the individual is king and where the illusion of separateness is the ultimate truth, to simply be – to expand their humanity and open their hearts. That in itself is important. That in itself is healing. That in itself is revolutionary in the most unassuming and unpretentious manner.

We are obligated to reconstruct our relationships with our family members and neighbors, with our allies and enemies, and most importantly with ourselves. We must rehabilitate our relationship with our life-enabling oceans and rivers, our forests and deserts, and with this phenomenon that is life.

These medicines, these mysterious plants and synthesized miracles of chemical engineering as one, can play a crucial role in enabling this process of reconciliation to materialize. Furthermore, the advent of the scientific revolution and the subsequent decline of monotheistic religions in Western societies are forcing many individuals to cope and face the ultimate life transition without a clear and solidified belief system, identifiable spiritual structure, or sufficient emotional support mechanism. Left to their own devices, individuals confronted with mortality are chained to an archaic and stereotypical vision of death; one that offers little solace and relief. Within this desperate existential gap and state of serious personal and global crisis, it is my strong belief that the substances in question have within them the capacity to revolutionize the psycho-emotional experience of death and thus transform our experience of life, with all that it entails.

The authentic human conquest is not one that is against death, the environment, or other members of the human family. It is neither a crusade against ignorance, greed, or the overcoming of our needs. It is a sacred internal pilgrimage towards a vision, an existence of comprehension and surrender, of humility and gratitude and of peace and reconciliation. For it is only by experiencing our infinite, shapeless, formless, and indeed boundless nature, the real nature of reality, that we can come to terms with, love and forgive, and accept and surrender to our own limited existence and perception as human beings.

*https://www.psymposia.com/magazine/israeli-defense-forces-ayahuasca-ptsd-1/*

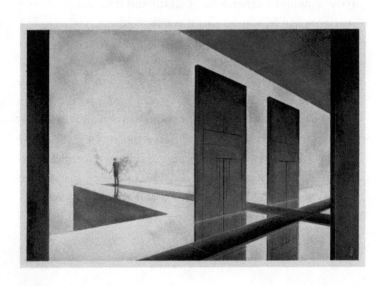

# THE SCREAMING ABYSS

## Psilocybin

As a result of reading *One Flew Over the Cuckoo's Nest* in my teens – and discovering that Ken Kesey wrote much of the novel under the influence of Psilocybin pinched from the state hospital where he was working – I developed a life-long dream to be in a clinical study with a psychedelic.

Later in life, I closely followed the various studies at Johns Hopkins, UCLA, and NYU and felt it would be an honor to be part of psychedelic history and help humankind. And so, I was accepted as a participant in the Phase I Psilocybin Pharmacokinetics Study, an FDA-approved clinical trial at the University of Wisconsin. The study intended to determine the pharmacokinetics of Psilocybin in support of Phase II and Phase III trials for people with incurable cancer.

After an application process and acceptance, I met my guides Dan and Karen through a series of four two-hour sessions. The meetings with my guides flowed smoothly. Sharing my story was mixed in with their own sharing from their lives. This helped cement a bond of trust that would serve me greatly as I progressed down into the pits of hell, which I had no idea I would soon be hitting. I was scheduled for three "dose days" where I would be administered Psilocybin – including the highest dose in this study. I entered all of this with the elation of a kid going off to summer camp mixed with a deep sense of honor to be part of such an important study.

My first dose was scheduled for August 27th, a beautiful late summer day. At the hospital I was given an IV, and my blood pressure was taken. Then I was escorted to the study room in UW's pharmacy building. Students were milling about and life seemed normal. I was about to do a high dose of Psilocybin. The surreal nature of this observation was beautiful to me.

Once settled into the comfy confines of Room 1010, the ceremony began. My guides did a quick check-in and hooked me up to an EKG. Then I was given my first dose of 99.8% pure Psilocybin – the entire Universe in a single capsule.

The whole setting of the session space was very calming and similar to a comfortable living room – complete with oriental rugs and trippy art on the walls. There was a cabinet filled with antipsychotic medication just in case someone went off the deep end, which was actually reassuring. At approximately 9 a.m. I took my first dose of 29 mg of Psilocybin. I took the dose with some anxiety and a lot of excitement.

All study participants were required to listen to an eight-hour mix of music. I laid back and put on eyeshades and headphones. George Winston began playing the piano in my ears. I hate George Winston, but I breathed and tried to relax.

After about twenty minutes, I felt the first wave. My body felt warm and then I felt nauseous. I never feel nauseous from mushrooms. I breathed deeply, but the nausea continued. I sat up and took the eyeshades and headphones off.

"I feel sick, like I might throw up," I said. I leaned over a bucket. I was sweating. The waves got more intense. I didn't like the direction this was going and started feeling concerned. I laid back down and went into the deepest and darkest journey of my life.

The next four hours were horrendous. I had never experienced such intensity, chaos, anxiety, panic, and insanity. There were no classic "visuals," only blackness mixed with impending and ever increasing internalized panic. I sat up again. "I think I'm having a bad trip," I said. "There is no bad trip; your experience is your experience. All is welcome," my guide said.

I laid back down and experienced more darkness, discomfort, and terror. I slid off the couch and ended up on the floor. While lying there, my body contorted and became unimaginable aliens, demons, and grotesque beings. There were no colors, only black and shades of black, darkness and despair.

Then came a moment when I saw myself "creating" all these entities. I was standing in an alleyway and realized that the demons were just a manifestation of my mind. It was merely a glimpse of insight, and for whatever reason I continued to torture myself with these horrendous, demonic images.

As I traveled through the pits of hell, a nurse performed EKGs, drew blood, and checked my blood pressure and my temperature. The amazing thing was these events became part of the journey. My experience was that I was on the sacrificial altar of humanity. My blood was a sacred elixir that was being taken by blood angels to the sacred chamber of lab analysis. My blood and body were serving mankind. In the midst of hell, I felt honored to be sacrificed for the sake of humanity. And I still do.

At one point I found myself trapped inside a black, rectangular box. Entities, creatures, and "things" were scurrying about the walls. A terrible stench mixed with these visuals. I was curled up in this box, and at this point one of the guides asked me, "Where are you?" I explained the situation. "See if you can find a light and flash it around – see what else is in there," she said. I found a headlight and put it on. With the light on I saw more nasty critters scurrying about.

Then I became one of "them" – a disgusting, pus-filled, cockroach-like creature that was expanding into the box. Then the box dissolved. I was back from the demonic, alien world, but still experiencing hell. The next hell realm was not mine, but felt like my father and my brother's hell. "I think I'm now taking one for the team," I said to my guides. This hell realm was now extending back through ages. It felt as if I was processing the "shit" of my ancestors. I was now about four hours into the experience.

At this point I had to use the bathroom. My bladder felt ready to burst. With guidance from Dan, I shuffled off to the bathroom. The bright lights and shininess felt strangely comforting. There was a photo of a lotus flower above the toilet. I stared at the lotus and watched it morph into female deities.

Now I was just "tripping." The walls were moving and the floor was melting. This felt good. I was on more familiar terrain, but I really needed to pee. The study required me to urinate into what is known as a "hat" – basically a large cup that resides in the bowl of the toilet. I sat down and began to pee. I stared at the floor as it shifted about and I felt a very strange sensation.

I looked down into the hat, and I saw that my scrotum was now floating in a pool of urine. I had peed so much that I filled the hat to the top and now my balls were happily floating about. "Dan! Dan! Can you come here? I need help!" I called. I heard Dan coming to the door. "What? What?" he said. "Can you come in here? I need help," I cried.

Dan entered the bathroom with a confused look on his face. I immediately dropped the bomb. "I peed so much my balls are now floating in my urine and I don't know what to do." I started to laugh. Dan started to laugh. "Well, I don't know what to do either," he said. We tag-teamed a paper towel cupping of my balls as I stood up. It is true love and dedication when your guide holds your urine soaked scrotum ever so gently in a wad of paper towels. It felt so good to laugh. I really thought I was out of the woods.

I shuffled back out and laid down on the couch. I curled up in the fetal position. I felt wiped out. I was still very much "in it," but I could feel the intensity tapering off. I remember thinking "I made it and I'm never, ever doing this again."

As I was lying there, a new wave came on. This one was equally as unpleasant as the earlier ones. I felt my brain "split." I was in the midst of a psychotic break, and I was witnessing this in slow motion as reality slipped away. I thought, "I'm going crazy. They will have to get a wheelchair to get me to the psych ward. I fucked up the study. I'm the first person to lose their mind during a study. Dan and Karen will be so pissed. I may have ruined the entire FDA approval process for Psilocybin. My kids! I'll never see my kids again in a normal state. I am crazy. I am getting crazier. Am I crazy? Yes…"

This went on for an hour as I sunk more and more into a delusional state of psychosis. Finally, I knew I had to sit up and break the bad news to Dan and Karen. And boy, were they going to be pissed! I sat up and slowly said, "I'm not doing good. I'm having a psychotic break."

Dan looked at me and exclaimed as he was bouncing in his chair, "That is awesome! Great work Steve! First journey of the dark soul and now you have gone crazy! Total breakdown of the OS! I am so happy for you!" Then Karen said, "Good work, Steve. Good work!"

I breathed and let all this in and thought to myself, "This is 'mind.' My mind! I created this!" I started to smile. I could see how my mind had manifested "crazy." I asked for my drum that I had brought for the session. Boom! Boom! Boom! Boom! I smiled and laughed. I got it. I got what I had created.

At the eight hour mark I was dismissed from Room 1010 and escorted back to my hospital room where I would spend the night. I ordered some dinner – a lovely chili-chicken stir fry.

My food arrived, and I sat down and this thought came in: "After the agony, dinner."

To be back in my body and eating a meal felt so normal and comforting. But I still hate George Winston.

Prior to dose number two, I had a meeting with my guides Karen and Dan. They asked the standard: "How have you been?" "I feel like I am in a cage," I said. "Tell us more," they replied. I always appreciated Dan and Karen's appreciation for my misery. They had me close my eyes, breathe deeply, and go inward.

"What do you see?" asked Karen. "I see a large wooden cage with metal bands suspended from a ceiling. I am inside, and there are small slots on each of the four sides. I'm being attacked from all four sides. I have a spear, and I am constantly going from one slot to the next, fending off the next attack," I said. "Where is the door? Can you get out?" Dan asked. "There is no exit. There is no way out…" I said. It was rather depressing to feel that. "During your journey tomorrow, we will revisit your cage and maybe you can hand the spears to me," Dan suggested.

It sounded like a great idea to lay down my weapons. I was slightly nervous about going back into the cage. The previous session was the most horrendous experience of my life, but I had complete trust in the medicine and the guiding of Dan and Karen. I also trusted my inner knowing and that I was in the study for a reason.

The next day the standard protocol applied. I checked in and was escorted to room 1010. This time my dose was 45 mg of pure Psilocybin. I took it and waited for the show to begin. There was fear and a sincere hope that this experience would not be as hellish.

The come-on was quick once again. This time it started with some colorful visuals. This was promising, but the beginning of the journey was chaotic. Hundreds of images were flashing by, though none seemed to make sense. I could feel edges of panic and anxiety, but I continued to breathe through it all.

At one point my cage appeared, three-dimensional and very colorful. It was twirling around and spinning. I realized I was outside the cage. I was just witnessing it. The cage was actually quite beautiful. It was no longer the dark, wooden, metal megalith of despair. I was watching it and had the feeling, "I no longer need you." Then it exploded into millions of bits of color.

"Where are you?" my guides asked me. "I was at my cage," I said. "Do you want to hand me your spear?" Dan asked. I replied back, "My cage exploded." There was some levity and much relief. The relief was not long-lasting though. Soon, I was hit with waves of discomfort. My body hurt. I felt anxious. I slid down to the floor and moaned. "Could someone please massage my back? I'm so sore," I pleaded. "Not now," Dan said. "Be with your experience." I could feel my desire to distract myself from my uncomfortableness, a major theme of my life.

What followed was a classic two-hour session of "looping." Looping is being stuck in a continual pattern of repetitive behavior or thought. It was very unpleasant and very disconcerting. I was sitting on the floor by Dan and Karen. I was stressed and panicky. "Why do I keep doing this to myself?" I asked. I could see how I was creating the discomfort and anxiety. I was slumped over breathing shallow, and then I would sit up, breathe, and say, "I'm doing this. I am creating this. It's so crazy. I need to stop." Then I would repeat this sequence over and over and over again.

"Why I am doing this? Why do I keep doing this?" I asked Karen. "You're in a thought loop. We are just here," she reassured me.

About halfway through this looping, four blocks of energy appeared around my shoulders. There were two on my front, and two on my back. When I slumped over, the energy stopped. When I sat up and breathed, the energy would start moving again. After two hours of this, I finally "got it." Sit up and breathe. Simple. But it seemed like I had to take the hard route to figure that out.

I was now about four hours in and was feeling somewhat "sane." My body felt sore, and I asked if I could receive bodywork at this point. I was very pleased to hear "yes."

What followed was subtle bliss. Karen spent about twenty minutes sitting behind me and gently and slowly moving my head around. Each movement was a different note of energetic frequency. It was very comforting and soothing. Then both Dan and Karen worked on me as I was lying down – total receiving in an altered stated.

After what felt like an hour into the bodywork, a small voice came out: "I feel like I need to cry." Soft tears began to fall, and then the dam broke. What followed was the most intense emotional purge of my life. Never have I experienced anything like the tidal wave of grief, anger, rage, tears, and sobbing that flowed through me. This grief was accompanied by yelling, screaming, and writhing.

Voices came out: "I was just a little fucking kid! You fucking monster! How could you do this to a little fucking kid! I just want a normal fucking father! I just wanted a normal fucking childhood! A normal fucking life! FUCK YOU! FUCK YOU! FUCK YOU! FUUUUUCCKKK…" I screamed. The rage, tears, and sadness were all directed at my father and brother. I thought I had addressed many of these issues previously but apparently not.

It is amazing what we can store in our bodies and psyches. It's all in there, and it wants nothing more than to be released. I felt a bizarre physical sensation of snot dripping down into my sinuses. This was followed by several epic nose blows. It felt great, like a sinus colonic. Having an emotional catharsis under the influence of Psilocybin has to be one of the more profound experiences that someone can go through. In the heightened state of Psilocybin, everything is amplified.

The session ended with me curled up in the fetal position. I felt spent. I was better on some levels, but experienced a persistent, low-level sadness in my soul and body. At one point I sat up and Dan and Karen were sitting on either side of me. I could feel their love. But I could feel my resistance to letting it in. I felt guarded and closed. I knew there was more work to be done.

After experiencing the flood of emotions from dose number two and the journey of the dark soul in dose number one, I was thinking, "I have experienced my darkness, my demons, and the underworld. I have purged my emotional blockage. I am ready to experience the divine. White light. Unity consciousness. Yes!" This was not to be. Even in writing this, I am flooded with tears.

Dose number three was the most intense, powerful, horrendous, terrifying, awful experience of my life. There is no way words can fully capture the horrifying intensity of this session. In the end, it was all worth it. I entered the most profound state that has forever changed my life.

Dose three was 59 mg. I received the largest dose of

Psilocybin ever administered in a published FDA study. For the uninitiated to Psilocybin dosing, this is a mega dose. The writer Terence McKenna dazzled his audiences with tales of doing what he called a "Heroic Dose" of 5 grams of dried mushrooms. I have been asked by many people "What does this equal in dried grams of mushrooms?" The answer: about 10 grams of dried mushrooms.

We went through the standard protocol: capsule, eye shades, headphones, lie down. And then…holy shit! There was really no ramp up. There was no warning. There was no gradual entry into hell. Within twenty minutes of ingesting the Psilocybin, I was shot directly into the infinite abyss of human suffering. I went quickly from lying down to sitting up. I took the eye shades and headphones off. Holy shit.

I was experiencing every person who had ever walked this Earth, who had ever suffered, every person currently living, every terrible thing that had ever happened to anyone, tortured, killed, lost a child, grieved. Every emotion tied to any human who suffered was being channeled through me. It was as if a fire hydrant of human suffering was going through me. As this was happening, I knew, "This is not me. This is not mine."

"Why me?" I called out. "Why am I experiencing this? Why am I carrying this burden? This is not mine." As this was happening, I thought I was screaming out a continuous wail. Later I learned that I wasn't, but my inner experience was that of a constant primal scream of suffering.

The intensity increased, and then at one point I saw an immense white hot circle lying before me. I felt myself fall into this abyss. Lining the abyss were thousands and thousands of souls screaming, writhing, all suffering as I fell downward into the pit.

This phase of dose three lasted about two hours, nonstop and relentless. At some point, I moved to the floor. I don't remember how I got there. I just remember somewhat "coming to" and out of the human suffering channel. The respite from that hell was soon followed by the next phase, my own suffering. This was not as horrendous as experiencing all of the suffering of humanity. It was just me. But it truly sucked.

Here I died, and died, and died again, hundreds of deaths of "Steve." I was parched, downtrodden, and beaten. I was a shell of a man suffering greatly. Then I would take a drink of water and fall over and die. I'd get back up, suffer, drink water, die, over and over again. At some point in this personal suffering as I was dying and writhing on the floor, Karen bent over and whispered, "Go deeper."

Bam! These were the perfect words at the perfect time. They assured me that I was okay on some level and that there was a deeper level to go to.

At about the four-hour mark, I sat straight up, breathed deeply, and witnessed the cycle of suffering that I was experiencing. It was an energetic swirl. It was happening in front of me – but I was no longer part of it. "It" was just "there."

What happened next is the most difficult part of the entire experience to fully convey in words for its depth and transformational power. I went from witnessing my swirl of suffering to a "place." I saw an infinite field of gray dust and a gray sky. Sitting in this dusty plain was a frail "boneman." Not a skeleton, but a boneman. The boneman was about two feet high sitting down. He sat cross-legged staring out at the infinite horizon. I saw him and then I became him. It was "I" that was sitting there. I was boneman.

Once I was boneman, I entered a stateless state. This stateless state was one of authority. I was pure awareness, but there was no awareness. I was pure consciousness, but there was no consciousness. There was a sense of pure wisdom and knowledge, but there was no wisdom or knowledge. It was a state of perfection, but there was no perfection. There was no desire. There was no emotion. There was no bliss. No oneness. No unity consciousness. There was nothing. This state was a perfect state. This state, which was not a state, was above all.

I came out of this place and shared a bit with Dan and Karen. I said that I felt I would need to do MDMA for PTSD from my human suffering session. I felt shell-shocked from that experience.

"Why don't you go back in?" Karen suggested. I closed my eyes and was instantly taken back to boneman.

I was sitting in pure presence, but there was no presence. And then boneman crumbled. He turned to dust. But "I" was still experiencing this stateless state. There was no object of "me."

My attention then shifted and I was now looking down on human suffering. Beneath me I could see the white ring to the portal of human suffering. There was no emotion, no feeling of compassion. It meant nothing. I then glanced in the other direction. I could "see" nirvana. It meant nothing.

At one point I experimented with dipping down into different levels of consciousness. I became a lion. I then became this noble, strong Danish warrior holding a spear and overlooking a large body of water. I could feel the full sense of this consciousness. It meant nothing.

What felt right was this state of high indifference. Ultimate authority of consciousness (that was not consciousness) that was above all levels of consciousness and unconsciousness. It was above the entire realm of what we can experience as humans.

I came out of it and was back on the couch in Room 1010. I looked around. I felt good, as if I were made of pure air. There was no density to me. I felt pure and clean. I have never felt better than that moment in my life.

Everything that I had suffered through to get to the state of boneman was worth it. It felt like those moments in that state were a culmination of my entire life. Everything that I had suffered through – the birth trauma, the suicide attempts, the divorces, the failures, were all paths to get me to boneman. To experience that state was the greatest gift and the most profound experience of my life.

It was more profound than the white light, unity consciousness, all-is-one experience I had on the 1,200 mcg of LSD. More profound than the spontaneous experiences of non-duality and the white light experience of my brother Mike. But even the immensity of this experience meant nothing.

It may sound nihilistic to be in such a state of indifference to the various modes of human consciousness. But the experience has left me a greater appreciation for all the nuances of life.

There is an intricately woven tapestry to our existence. A tapestry of pain, suffering, grief, joy, love, bliss, ecstasy, and thousands of variations of these potential aspects of being human. None of them are better or worse than the other. They are all just "there" – there for us to experience, to feel. To be alive is to embrace it all, and not put any meaning on any of it. Every experience is a fleeting moment of time. "It" is there in one moment, and in the next moment it is gone. What is left is the illusion of memory.

Where we get lost is in the stories that we create. The meaning that we assign to experiences. What I am learning is that nothing means anything, and conversely, everything means something. Without meaning there is no story to an event, occurrence, or memory. Our ego-mind assigns meaning based on past experiences, filters, distortions, and lies. Meaning comes through a story – what we attach to an event. We assign meaning to everything, but it means nothing.

Meaning is a self-manifested story constructed from the illusion of time. There is no past. There is no future. The past and the future are simply illusions of our mind. "You are a terrible, ugly person" has no more meaning than "You are the most amazing, beautiful person in the world." It's not until we attach meaning to something that it exists as a story – a false story with no true meaning. Only a manifestation of the mind.

We needlessly suffer based on attached meaning. The false reality we have created from thousands of stories that have no meaning. If we can dissolve to a state of no "I," there is no suffering, no attachment, no seeking, and no searching. We simply exist in a state of present moment awareness where all is as it should be – the perfection of existence in the moment. From this place, our true nature (for every one of us) of pure being, pure awareness, pure love and compassion shines. Nothing means anything… just be.

Within all of this comes a realization that every one of us in this very moment (even as you read this) is awakened, enlightened, and in a state of perfection. You are already "there." It only takes a perceptual shift, a breath of awareness, a flash of realization to discover the illusion of life.

The beautiful thing is in that moment of realization you fully understand that being awakened or enlightened means nothing. It's the great cosmic giggle. We all want it, we all seek it, and then in a flash we realize we all already have it, and once you have it – it means nothing…HA! The perceptual shift of realization.

For me a great metaphor is this scene: You are running late for something. Trying to rush out the door but you cannot find your car keys! Where are they? You are running through the house searching, looking, and beating yourself up because you don't know where they are. "How can I be so stupid!? I'm going to be late! People will be upset. I'm such a loser," you think. Then you stop, pause, breathe and allow a slight glance to the right and down, and you realize, in a moment of presence, that this whole time you have been holding the keys in your hand. They have been right "there" all along. It just took a pause and a perceptual shift and BAM! What you were seeking, you held.

Enlightenment is like that. EVERYTHING we seek is like that. It's right "there." You already have it and you have always had it. In this moment and in every moment of your existence you are complete, whole, perfect and awakened.

In regards to heroic doses, large doses, and shamanic doses, I feel it is important to deemphasize the dose factor. It's not about dose size – bigger is not necessarily better. I know people who have had profound, life-changing experiences from 3 grams.

I think what is most important for any journey is your willingness and readiness to dive in, to be open to whatever presents itself. My intention going into my sessions was a simple – "I am ready to receive whatever I need for my life at this moment." I was apparently ready for the journey of the dark soul. I think what I experienced would have happened even if the dosage was half as much.

Also, there were a number of synchronistic events that led up to and were part of the three month journey (one dose per month). One week prior to my first dose I attended a three day holotropic breathwork workshop with Stan Grof. The seeds of birth trauma were planted. After the first dose, I heard my birth story from my mother for the first time in my life. What I discovered was that I was a breech baby. The doctors first attempted to manually flip me around, but the pain was so great for my mom that she was put under general anesthesia. I was then "extracted" vaginally with broken ribs and then carted off to the nursery where they were unaware that I had broken ribs. If you read Stan Grof's BPM II stage, it fits perfectly with my first dose experience. This was a huge piece in the puzzle of Steve.

I think a huge factor in where I went on my journey was my setting. I was in the safest and most trusted place possible to go deep and into the darkest recesses of my psyche. The trust I had with my guides and with the medicine allowed me to completely let go into the dark abyss of my soul/psyche. And this trust in the medicine and my guides is what kept me coming back – I knew there was deep work to be done and I knew I was in good hands. I was committed to take this journey to wherever it took me.

My three doses were a primary release of the trauma I was holding since birth. What I experienced as a new born was a horrific and excruciatingly painful birth followed by abandonment. What I experienced during the study was the release of that. And with that release my life has forever changed. The filters of depression and anxiety that I had my entire life are gone. I had wondered all my life, "What is wrong with me?" Coming to the realization of my birth experience and the ensuing release of the emotions, suffering, pain, and grief has brought a new Steve to the world.

One thing I want to reiterate is that my Psilocybin guides, and the entire staff from UW-Madison, were impeccable in their guidance and in allowing me to go into these hell realms. They trusted the medicine and they trusted my own inner strength and willingness to go deep, and then to go even deeper. I had to go there… I had to release the suffering… and with that release was my own personal freedom and joy.

*https://www.psymposia.com/magazine/largest-dose-psilocybin-fda-study-1/*

# THE KEY

## Ibogaine

Opioid addiction. I had always heard that to kick it meant go through hellish sickness and maddening withdrawal. Even once complete you would always still crave the drugs. I had been on methadone and then suboxone maintenance for almost four years for a pain pill addiction that turned into a ten bag a day heroin habit. I was determined to get off all of it. To be free.

My taper with the maintenance meds went very slowly but when I got to 2 mg of suboxone a day, I hit a wall. During the years of my taper I started a meditation practice, but it wasn't until the "wall" that I went into the practice with an intention. My question to the Universe: "How do I finish this process and free myself from this substance?" Then, one day while I was meditating by a creek the answer came to me. There was a plant medicine out there to treat this. I immediately went inside and consulted Google. Within minutes I found Iboga.

A medicine derived from a plant! Bingo. It is claimed that you take this medicine and enter a dreamlike state where a guide takes you on a journey. Meanwhile your body detoxes and you don't go through withdrawal. The only problem was the shit was illegal in the U.S. My search for a qualified provider began. It didn't take me long until I found two men who had trained with the shamans in West Africa and were conducting detoxes.

I contacted these guys and they gave me a list of requirements before treatment. First, they needed my backstory. I also needed liver panels to make sure I could process the medicine and a note from my doctor that stated my heart was okay. The men also requested that I start taking a series of supplements. The date was set for Halloween night. I was hell-bent on trying Ibogaine, and with the help of the Universe I somehow managed to come up with the few thousand dollars for the treatment.

I went with my boyfriend and met my shamans. They were jovial and chatty. After a grocery run the ceremonies began. We went to a local park and they conducted a ceremony, asking the Earth for permission. We then went back to our space where I was given my first test dose. A bath was drawn for me and it was filled with flowers and herbs. I was told to get in the water and confess my sins out loud and wash myself each time. To make sure the ritual was complete, when I finished, my shaman chewed up some seeds, spit them on the carpet and read them. The seeds spoke: I was ready to journey.

Within ten minutes of taking my first real dose, I began to feel my Root Chakra open up and vibrations came from beneath my feet. My loved one kissed me goodbye and left me with the shamans. Painted in traditional Bwiti ceremony paint, the two men stood above me. Not soon after the vibration started, I began hearing what could only be described as jungle music. Drumming and chanting. This was coming from inside of me. Then, lift off!

I felt like I was inside of a rocket ship racing towards the stars. I felt higher than I had ever been. In moments, I broke through some sort of crystalline glass structure and was floating in blackness. The panic began to set in as I didn't know what the fuck was happening or what I had just signed up for. As soon as the panic started, a tiny slit opened in the blackness. A large green eye shined through and an elf-like creature that reminded me of a miniature Peter Pan reached in and crawled into the blackness with me. It didn't speak to me with words but telepathically and with body language. I felt safe and when it reached for me, the scene changed.

I was in the crystalline room again. Each crystal had an image from my life. The guide reached for me again and took me into a scene of where I was a baby and my grandfather was reaching for my finger. I don't know if I actually physically sobbed on the outside, but inside I cried out of pure gratitude for being able to see this. It went on for hours and hours like this but to me it felt like months. Time eventually disappeared as I traveled in and out of the scenes of my life, both good and bad. The guide never let me stay anywhere too long.

Toward the end of my journey a strange test began. First, I was shown a toy rocking horse. I was shown every single component to what went into creating this horse. Everything down to the photons that created the DNA that created the seed that created the tree that created the wood. This continued for all the tools that were used to make the rocking horse and then it began for the people that chopped the wood, that shipped the wood, that built the horse, that sold the horse. It showed me their ancestors, their DNA. I felt like I was in some sort of mental marathon.

It was exhausting and dizzying, and I was being quizzed.

While I was being quizzed I was being forced to run up and down strands of DNA. The ultimate answer was me understanding what the fear of God is. An infantile understanding of the interconnection and complexity that is the creator and the creation. That is all things. With me coming to this realization, an understanding happened between me and my guide and everything began to move very slowly. A black skeleton key was taken from me. A key that I didn't even know I had inside of me. I was told it was my addiction and I would never be able to find this key again. That I was free.

I started to slowly wake up out of this to find one of my shamans playing an instrument at the foot of my bed – an ngombi harp. I vaguely remember him playing this with his teeth. I faded in and out. When I finally came to, I felt dreamy and ungrounded. Like part of my consciousness was floating above my body. In my entire life, I don't think I'd ever been as quiet as I was in the days following this experience. Processing what I had experienced took me months. It's important to note that I experienced zero withdrawal.

I did this on October 31st. Halloween night is my anniversary. I have been clean and have never craved an opioid since. By the grace of God and the help of Ibogaine I have been freed.

# LIFE IS BUT A DREAM

## Psilocybin

Most of my life, I had struggled with depression, anxiety, and seriously low self-esteem. I had a chaotic and sad childhood with little to no support. I lived and thrived on the "brainwashed" side of society; completely immersed in reality TV, gossip magazines, trash music, and having total faith in our government. I lived in fear: fear of not succeeding, fear of going to Hell, fear of not being loved, and fear of not having validation from friends, family, and co-workers.

In the midst of a severely toxic relationship and being enlisted in the Marine Corps, I had made a friend who introduced me to the Law of Attraction, meditation, conspiracy theories, and energy work. My ego and programmed beliefs fought her every step of the way, yet it had still ignited a flame in my heart. The seed was planted. I wanted to learn more and explore the other side of the wall I had worked tirelessly to build up.

Fast forward to a year post-military, post-divorce, and somewhat "awakened." It was my first time ever using Psilocybin mushrooms. I had only ever smoked weed before, and my knowledge of psychedelics was limited. My boyfriend had experienced Psilocybin mushrooms a handful of times, all within a ceremonial setting. For the first few months of our relationship, he had been slowly introducing me to pieces of his own collective experiences and informative speeches by Alan

Watts and Terence McKenna.

I had set my intention. I wanted to learn how to let go of my ideas, anger, and past heartaches. I wanted to know what it felt like to be at peace in my heart. I fasted for a few hours prior, and my boyfriend provided some fruit and orange juice for the trip. The apartment was cleaned and smudged, music playlists ready, incense burning, and intentions were set.

My boyfriend, his roommate, and I, all sat with 5 grams in the palm of our hands. I watched everyone chase them with orange juice, grimacing at the grainy, Earthy taste. I felt nervous and unsure. My boyfriend saw this and said, "Baby you don't have to do anything. Only if you feel it's right." Here it was, my first test, fear ever present and screaming in my face. I decided to "go in" and finished eating mine within seconds.

The first thirty minutes or so had minimal effect. I got the common symptoms: sweaty palms, tight chest, minor nausea, and anxiety. I breathed through this and headed down the hallway to my boyfriend's room. Upon entering, a dim lamp partially lit his room, and soft new age music played. I felt euphoric. I felt like moving and stretching, as I also felt too big for my body. At this point, I understood how yoga is beneficial. I also understood that I felt too big for my body because I am not my body. I am not my skin, or my fingers, or my hair.

I lied on the floor, tired, sweating, and eyes watering. My body felt heavy and awkward, and my breathing was shallow. Mandalas bloomed across the ceiling in blues and greens and I noticed that their shape and speed had changed with each song playing through the speakers. The music had affected my visuals and each song brought about certain emotions.

At one point, I had the thought that I might be dying. This thought spurred a perpetual list of things that could go wrong. The dark parts of the room grew darker, and the clothes hanging in the closet started to fill out and form bodily shapes. My fear was manifesting my reality. I suddenly remembered my intention and all I could do was breathe and accept my "impending death." And just like that, the room brightened, my body felt lighter, and I had a little more energy.

I can only assume that I had an ego death. I came to understand that my inner reality was directly affecting my outer reality; just as it does in daily life. I had realized that a bad trip isn't bad. It is only a confrontation of self. I had to face my fear of losing control, I had to get lost, and then I had to let go and accept in order to come out of it. "This wave has to crash."

I looked at my phone to see what time it was and I saw code. The numbers looked like code from the movie Predator. I also realized that the phone in general was a foreign thing to me. It didn't make sense. I knew that somewhere in my mind I understood how to use it, but I just couldn't get my brain to connect to my fingers.

I walked back into the hallway, eager to tell my boyfriend what I had experienced. His roommate, who was generally a negative person and tripping only for the high aspect, was lying on the couch, staring intensely at his phone. A garbage reality show was on TV, and the living room itself was a whole other world.

The voices on the TV sounded like demonic gibberish. I

turned to say something to my boyfriend, who was looking at me with shock. "Do you hear that too?" he asked. I nodded and walked over to his roommate. The living room looked plastic and fake, like a life-size doll house. I tried talking to his roommate, who only stared at his phone and shook his head, as if to tell me to leave him alone. It wasn't until later that I learned he had heard the voices on the show just fine, and he thought my boyfriend and I were demons. The fake glossiness of the room reflected his state of mind; he was closed off, afraid, and angry.

Throughout the night, minutes seemed like hours, and magic was happening at every turn. I'd kept my distance from his roommate, and focused on my visuals. Sanskrit shimmered down the hallway walls and floor. My fingers created ripples as I dragged them through the air. When I looked in the mirror, I saw the faces of everyone I loved flash over my own, ending on my own face aging dramatically. I shook my head and closed my eyes until it stopped.

I recalled my mother, whom I have a tumultuous relationship with. I immediately saw her as a child. I had nothing but love and compassion for her, and for everyone who had ever hurt me. I saw everything and everyone through God's eyes. My eyes were the same eyes through which God see, as I and everyone else is created as a God.

When I looked at my boyfriend, his body aged. Muscles, tendons, and veins would show through his aging skin, and I had another understanding of our impermanence. At times, his nose and facial hair along with the hair on his head would spike out like the human characters of Pokémon. The shape of the cartoonish hair would change with every blink of my eyes, until I decided it was enough; then he would just be a beautiful human – the MOST beautiful human.

At one point, my boyfriend grew frustrated with his roommate's negativity and this frustration was creating a reality for him. I heard him yell at his roommate on the balcony for disrespecting the medicine, and as I looked up, I saw him throw his water bottle. He had his shirt off, and his skin was cherry red and glossy with sweat. He was breathing heavily and his eyes turned black. I decided to allow him to go through this. "He needs this." I thought, and I took my dog outside to pee.

While outside, I was too concerned with watching the magic of nature to worry about what was happening in the apartment. I saw the Chi of life flowing bright green through the tree, to its roots, connecting to the soles of my feet. I felt the powerful presence of the tree and asked its permission to share that plot of grass. I sat and watched the stars bounced off of each other, following a sacred grid which aligned them. My dog got little attention, as she kept shapeshifting. First, I'd see a creature with hair and teeth, then, as she walked across the yard, she slowly transformed into a genderless, hairless being, crawling over the grass. I shook my head and decided I was done with that, and she was back to being a dog.

At a certain point, my boyfriend came walking down the stairs. I asked him if he was alright, to which he replied, "I have to be." Then we went back inside. He explained to me that he was lost. The room was stretched and the ceiling was so high, he could barely see it. He said that he saw me by the door, but I looked so far away and he wasn't sure if I was me. He felt that the chaos he was feeling spun him into a chaotic reality, and it wasn't until I presented the question, "Are you alright?" that he was able to pull out of it. I had to present the question so that he could find the answer.

I decided to try and talk to his roommate. I wanted to tell him that I loved him and how perfect everything is. I sat at his feet, while he sat on the couch and stared down at me. He told me I was disrespectful, and that when I was bouncing around and expressing my excitement, it was infiltrating "his space." As he was condemning me, I watched this black tar-like shadow grow and climb out from under him. It covered the couch and the wall behind him, and I started to get scared. I already felt bad about being "too happy." I was buying into his anger, into HIS reality. And as soon as I started to believe him, the gooey shadow started to cover my toes. I refused to go into his world, so I talked to him as a child – one who needed unconditional love and guidance. I called him sweetie and apologized, and attempted to make him laugh. When he finally laughed, the darkness disappeared and the room was brighter.

I couldn't believe it. How strong manifestation is. All night, I was being shown what your thoughts and feelings do to your outside world. I was being shown how destructive I've been to myself.

Eventually, my boyfriend and I retired to his room. We laid in his bed, with him behind me, arm over my waist. We both had different, but similar visuals, yet we felt the same thing – an infinite and unconditional love for each other. For me, the room was a smoky haze of glitter, light, and color, and the walls were covered in jungle flowers and plants. We both saw our bodies as one body and laughed and cried in awe of how connected we were. There weren't enough times or ways to tell each other we loved one another. It was the most beautiful and innocent spiritual connection I had ever felt.

I've tripped a few times since then. By myself, with friends, micro-dosing, and large doses. I've had equally significant yet different experiences each time. Mushrooms have changed my whole existence. The day after my first trip, I cut my cable, stopped listening to the radio, stopped celebrating holidays, and stopped participating in major consumerism. I'm a far better being. I'm saved. I'm love. I'm awake.

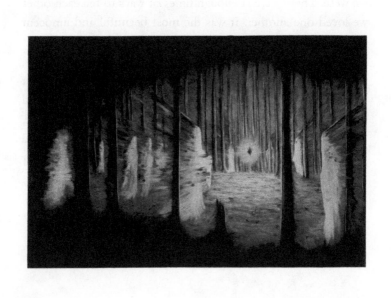

# THE RESISTANCE HAD TO END IF I WAS TO BEGIN

## San Pedro

There is talk of a calling that one receives. I firmly believe in this. When I look back at each and every step from my past to present it seems like a perfectly choreographed dance of lessons, interactions, ups, downs, and everything in between. I feel as though I've reached the apex of a peak and can now finally look back and see the entire path and its intricate meandering route. This is a testament to now, I suppose, for to be able to look back at life in general and have no regrets, just awe and wonder at how it took each step to get here, is something special. And I'm fully in love with here, with now, with life, and ultimately with me.

It was June when I had taken my first step into the world of shamanism and plant medicines. It was a necessary step, but somehow it wasn't the huge plunge that I may have been hoping for. Somewhere in me I was still resisting, still holding on, and still trying to outsmart the process. Within a month or two of returning from that adventure I felt the pull again. Life wasn't all that perfect at home and there was this feeling of, "I need to make a shift, and something has to change." This time it was San Pedro, also called Huachuma (although Don Howard explained it was definitely different from San Pedro) that called me. When you know it's time you just know, so in January I booked my journey.

Many things in my life were coming to a head. Anxiety, heartache, and an overall sense of constantly living in limbo had become a large part of my waking life. Something had to shift. My parting note to life in Canada was the great Heraclitus quote, "No man ever steps in the same river twice, for it is not the same river and he is not the same man." I knew there was a change on the horizon; I just couldn't have imagined how dramatic it would be.

Through taxis, airplanes, and buses I rapidly ended up at the SpiritQuest Sanctuary outside of Iquitos, Peru. It felt as natural as could be. Of course there were still some nerves as to what might come but overall it couldn't have gone smoother.

We were to partake in three ceremonies over the seven-day retreat, each ceremony having a feel or theme to it. The first was water, incorporating a sense of levity and birthing. The second would be Earth, in which Don Howard alluded to the fact that there may be some heavy times and if need be we'd have to acknowledge and sit with those feelings. The third and final would be air, in which we'd have a chance to connect beyond our Earthly confines and go into the astral realm. I wondered how three ceremonies with the exact same medicine could have three very different effects. Huachuma was also described as hitting one with a feather rather than a hammer. Let me tell you, it was one very very heavy and slow feather. It's tough to describe this in words and metaphor. This medicine is known as a heart opener and the mesada, or initiation, is an introduction to the jaguar spirit to eliminate our fear. The experience couldn't have hit either of these points more perfectly.

In the past, I always tried to be the recorder. I tried to take the experience, outsmart it, and create wordplay to describe it and bring it back to others. This time, things became truly ineffable. I'll be writing about this and thinking about it for my entire life, but there is a core to it that will never be described properly. It must be experienced rather than relayed.

The first ceremony (water) began. Each individual was called up to the altar, known as the Mesa. Two fingers on each hand plugged into the edges of the table. Don Howard cleansed and protected us with his mapacho smoke and rattles. When the music stopped we drank a not too bitter brew from a large cup. Once the medicine was down it was just a waiting game. What would happen next?

For me that first session was quite light. My intention going in was to be an open vessel to the Universe, ready to accept love. I also aimed at connection to all and a sense of safety. Before I drank, Don Howard said to me, "You're here for a reason aren't you brother? It's all about love and connection here, you are safe." With that, he had read my mind and I knew I was in good hands. It was the first of many mystical experiences and I hadn't even drank the brew yet.

Almost immediately after drinking we gathered our belongings and headed out for the day for a boat ride down the river. I listened to my headphones to drown out the motors and it began to get quite beautiful, everything slightly enhanced. The music became an impressive soundtrack to the beauty of life in the Amazon. The entire time I was processing what was going on, trying to gauge it, trying to hold on. Well, my ego was trying to hold on I suppose. I felt a sense of buoyancy, but still I couldn't let go.

We visited a tribe. Smiling faces and joy were all around us. Children with the best smiles I'd ever seen. We watched a ceremonial song and dance and were then free to wander about.

Again, this first session was not quite as deep as I might have imagined. I wouldn't let it get too deep. There were some very beautiful moments, but overall I began to wonder if this was the right path for me.

The boat ride home was quite glorious. I chose the ideal music for the trip and as the sun set I started to catch a glimpse of what this medicine could be. By the time we returned to the ceremonial hut, known as the maloca, I was all but back to myself. There were others who were directly plugged in that night, but for me it had already faded to a mere whisper. The first ceremony was complete and I still had many questions.

That night I couldn't sleep at all. I had the most excruciating headache. It felt like things were being shifted and torn out in there, like long strands of pain were being dragged across my mind. I didn't know what to make of this but it seemed like an important step. Something had to be rewired if I were to continue.

The second ceremony (Earth) was still filled with the unknown for me. I hadn't gone deep enough in the first ceremony so I didn't know what to expect. Through the same ceremony, we drank our medicine and again headed out for the day. This time I knew immediately it was going to hit me harder.

There was that sense of levity, but there was something deep and heavy intertwined in there as well.

Another glorious boat ride. Music had never sounded so perfect to me. This time we went on a hike for about forty minutes. It felt good to move, to be in the jungle, to feel very much connected with nature. Still, my mind held on. I was resisting but beginning to lose that battle. We ended up at a clearing with a small pond for swimming. Through the circumstance and having recently had my back tattooed, I couldn't go for a swim, so I stood and watched.

There was a moment when the rain began to fall and the sun was shining on the water – the staccato of light, reflection, and ripple. There was a moment there that still feels as though it's reverberating through eternity.

I felt stuck, physically and mentally. I was at an impasse and something had to give. We went back to another small clearing and the tribe was about to do a ceremonial dance. At this point, everything got extremely heavy for me. I felt the Earth pulling me down, engulfing me. It was eternal and immense and I knew not what to do. Every negative thought began to fill my head, "This is bullshit, look at us, just a bunch of drugged up foreigners in the jungle. This is scheisterism not shamanism. Fuck it, I'm never doing this again."

On and on these thoughts went. I felt heavier and heavier. It was the closest to death I think I've ever felt. I cannot describe it better than that. It was a death of sorts. There was a part of me, or my ego, that had to die. The resistance had to end if I was to begin and so I let go. I let the medicine finally take hold in full effect. I surrendered and accepted what was given. From there everything became magnificent.

The tribe did a ceremonial song and dance and with each moment I began to feel my power return. We hiked back to the boats and that boat ride, man that was something else. I watched the most miraculous sunset set to music and my heart was so wide open at this point. I'd never felt such an immense sense of calm, of peace, of love and belonging. Returning to the maloca we partook in more ceremony. This time I was plugged in. This time I was beginning to get it.

There are moments that are beyond words. As Terence McKenna would say, they are "un-Englishable." From here on in that rang so very true, but nonetheless I'll give it a try.

The third ceremony (air) was filled with excitement for me. I had a sense of what was to come. The fear had subsided and all that remained was wonder and awe. This time, we drank and then immediately went for a hike. It was a matter of minutes before I was tuned in and vibrating with an energy of connection that I cannot describe. The jungle was me and I was the jungle, a shared experience by almost everyone in the group. The trees were whispering all around us and the Earth was breathing. Yes… breathing. I would sit and watch and it was undeniable. Everything else would be perfectly still and I'd see a small pocket of Earth calmly inhaling and exhaling. It was beautiful.

And that's what I was told of Huachuma – it's a clarifier. It doesn't alter what is there; it just allows us to truly see what is going on all around us all of the time. This time it was so very different. I had plugged in completely. There was no resistance on my part.

My intention for this day was, "Accept what it given. Respect all things," and this mantra rang so very true for the entirety of the process. Again, there are moments which I cannot describe. I was given the knowledge that the Universe is infinite and eternal and at the core of it is all love. To know this rather than think it or theorize it, this is something different. The hang-ups and fears that we create, they are so very bizarre. All that we are here to do is be the best person we can possibly be. The Universe wants me to fully experience it through the best possible Cohen imaginable. For that's what we are, the Universe playing hide and seek with itself and when this incarnation ends we get to go back to the whole and repeat and repeat and repeat. I love the analogy of Alan Watts, the idea that we are all waves in the ocean. When one wave crashes it is not sad, the ocean remains the ocean and is not individuated into single waves coming or going.

A sense of strength and calm continued to grow in me throughout the day. Eventually we made our way to the sky deck, a platform at the highest point for as far as the eye could see. This was where most of us got stuck in time, or stepped out of time perhaps. It was just pure awe and bliss, staring at the sky just above the canopy of the jungle. There are no words to describe this, but I do know that most of us had a shared experience there. It was difficult to move, for I didn't want to disturb the perfection of "now."

At one point I laid back on the warm concrete. Eyes closed, the rain began to hit me. It was total synesthesia. Each drop was a staccato burst of light on my body. I could see each point where it hit me and touch, sound, sight… it all melded into one perfect harmony. I don't know how long we were up at the skydeck, but it felt like eternity. It feels like I'm still there to some degree.

Eventually we began to make our way down to the maloca. This time I was still so astoundingly plugged in. I would sit with eyes closed and see very clearly the energetic pattern of what was going on around me. It was so much brighter inside my head with eyes closed than it was outside with eyes open: vibratory patterns of purple and green on a matte black background. Just pure bliss and connection. It felt as though my head had opened at the top and the dome of the Universe was one and the same. I was everything and everything was me. The edges between everything had completely dissolved. The separation of self had completely obliterated. I was surfing the cosmic sea and it was so very very perfect.

At one point, Don Howard approached me from behind, but even with my eyes closed I could still see him in perfect detail. He crouched over me, his being arching over the view of the eternal and it was so very gentle and tender and loving.

There isn't a doubt in my mind that he was viewing straight into my core, seeing all that I was seeing.

The ceremony eventually ended, but my journey was still going strong. Some of us remained in the maloca for quite some time, watching as the candles burnt out one by one. There was a part of me that watched that last candle flicker and dance, a part of me that fully believed that when that candle went out so would all else. I would be extinguished and return to the ocean, my wave cresting and falling, and perhaps this happened to some degree.

Something amazing shifted over these three ceremonies. Every little fear I had ever had, I left there in the Amazon. There was this sense of calm and warmth that pervaded everything. There was an overwhelming love and awe for existence. My head and my heart had both been opened so wide that there was no chance they would ever begin to close. For those of you that know me, well, I'm sure you've seen this in me. The shift was so very real. There was a glow to life that I'd never experienced before and each interaction became more exciting and important. Each connection was a new opportunity and adventure.

For the first few days I'd wake up worried that this feeling might be fleeting, that it might fade, but I'm glad to say this has not been the case. I've truly returned from the river a different man. Suddenly everything in life is so very exciting, and the perspective shift, man, it's something else. All of those hang-ups and forms of resistance, they're all just gone. Fear is such an anchor and I've become untethered. Without a doubt, this was the most important month of my life and the reverberations of which will be felt for the rest of my days.

There is far more to this story, but I feel as though this has been a small taste of what I'm thinking and feeling. It's tough to describe that which is beyond words but I've given it a try. That feather of Huachuma, it hit so very slow and so very heavy, an impact which I didn't even see coming. Now my life is virtually unrecognizable. I feel so very loved and cared for by everyone around me. Connections which I may have ignored due to fear and the unknown, they are springing up at every turn – the community I've always dreamed of has been sitting there for me to grasp all along. The life I've wanted to lead, I'm getting to lead it now. I have said aloud many a time over the past few weeks, "This is the life I get to lead?" I'm in utter awe of the Universe and my place in it. Yes, this is the life I get to lead; this is the life I will navigate with an open heart and a calm mind.

Accept what is given.

Respect all things.

I have so much gratitude for life and connection and all of those who have played a role in this.

Thank you.

# IMPERMANENT IMMORTALITY

## DMT

Eyes closed and lying on a beanbag chair, I was launched into the astral realm filled with infinite mandalas and ever-changing fractal imagery. The nature of the three-dimensional space we're used to had been elevated to the nth degree. The g-force was so extreme it actually projected out from inside my core. If this isn't hyperspace, I'm not sure what is. Welcome to my Saturday night.

It was a quiet Saturday night in May and after taking a short hiatus from psychedelics, I decided it was time to experience DMT once again. The thing about DMT is that no matter how experienced I might be in any psychedelic substance, nerves still creep into my spine whenever I'm about to take the plunge. Because of the unpredictability of DMT, you'll never know what you'll be encountering. Entering the unknown has always given me an uneasy feeling in my stomach because I know intuitively how deep I'm about to go.

Everything was set; I was on a balcony lying on a bean bag chair while listening to a recording of Om chanting from Tibetan monks. Nervousness was still present but there was no turning back. I lit the incense and set my intention for the journey: to learn about our universe. After four deep hits of the substance, everything faded into darkness. I closed my eyes and

and dropped my head back... it had begun.

I was propelled into a universe of ever changing mandalas. They were all spherical, multidimensional, and beautiful in every way possible. Within the mandalas were characters that were constantly transforming into symbols and other forms of art that I couldn't recognize. Jester spirits appeared and multiplied by the thousands right in front of my eyes. My body was flying in and through all the sacred spheres. The jester spirits also claimed a large spiritual presence, forming a force field. At one point, I even became one of the mandala spheres itself, indistinguishable from my body. Time seemed irrelevant; I was fully in the moment, in total awe.

Although this was a place I'd never been to, it felt eerily familiar. At that moment I thought, what if this was the place where we go when we die? What if I'm dying right now? What if I'm really experiencing death? I felt my body tighten and immediately reminded myself to let go. What's the worst that could happen? If this was death, it might not be so bad after all. I started to find comfort in death. I started to find peace within, no matter what was happening. I was free.

As I let go, I felt myself diving deeper and deeper into hyperspace. The Om chants playing in my ears seemed to be getting louder without any adjustments to the volume. As the monks chanted "Ommmmm," the sound wave of the Om itself formed a powerful mandala and pierced right through my heart. It was so intense that I wanted the chanting to stop badly. It felt as if my consciousness was an overfilled balloon that was about to burst at any second. Who knew the simple sound of Om could possess so much power? As fear crept in, I continued to remind myself to let go.

Suddenly, at the corner of my eye emerged a burning sun. It was so bright that I could barely look directly at it, even with my eyes completely shut. My physical body was quickly warming up as the heat rays touched my skin. The energy was so intense that it was impossible to face it directly without being blinded. The sun moved from one corner to another in light speed until I felt the presence of entities looking down upon my body, as I found myself lying down on an operating table. What the hell was I doing on an operating table?

Four entities appeared from the top of my view. Somehow, I understood intuitively that they were intelligent beings. They also carried a mysterious, yet trollish energy that made me feel quite uncomfortable. I knew they were operating on my body, but I didn't know if they were friend or foe. I had no choice either way. Suddenly, I felt waves of smoke blown on my body. They were performing a ritual. As the smoke wrapped around me, my warmed body started to cool down from the heat of the burning sun. I could physically smell the essence of the smoke and feel the coolness flooding my body, mind, and consciousness. It was healing me. It was a cleanse. It was intense.

As the sounds of Om continued to burst through my eardrums and into my consciousness, the entities continued the healing. My vision became so clear that I could see the millions of fractals and sacred geometries that were flooding the remaining spaces the entities didn't occupy. Although I had no control over anything in this realm, it felt oddly comforting.

Instead of always wanting control, there was a beauty in just being a witness to watch things unfold without ego or judgment.

Slowly, I felt the Om sound losing the intense power it once carried. The sacred geometry all around also began to consolidate piece by piece, no longer dancing in its sacred fractal arrangements. I knew at this point it was time to return to my home dimension. A sense of relief dawned on my psyche, as this was by far one of the most intense DMT trips I'd ever journeyed. The vivid imagery started to become plain; the 9th dimensional plane compressed and became flat. I felt gravity again.

I opened my eyes and was in absolute shock. I questioned how I could be in hyperspace just seconds ago and now back in the beanbag chair? I also questioned the nature of the Universe and the implications this experience brought forth. Although my rational brain understood the scientific processes of self-induced DMT release, my heart could not fathom the depth of this incredible chemical. This is an incredibly powerful tool.

After the experience, the thoughts of an impermanent immortality had consumed my mind. The mandalas I had witnessed were continuously expanding and inverting in a boundless fashion. As everything had no beginning or end, it was the true meaning of infinity. I had the realization that there was no such thing as birth or death, as we are all energies flowing in and out of existence, always here, or never there. This was the message from the mandalas. This was the lesson the Universe taught me. This was what my third eye needed to see.

Still sitting on the beanbag chair, I was shaken and

overwhelmed by the powerful imagery that transcended my soul. Although I was still slightly dazed from the drug, I had never felt so alive. I carried a sense of confidence which ensured me that no matter what happened, everything would be okay. Without hesitation, I lit another stick of incense, set my intention for the second time. And off I went, back into the stars, into the realms of the infinite, into an impermanent immortality.

# TRANSFORMATION THROUGH DEATH AND REBIRTH

## LSD + MDMA + Ketamine

The night started off great, spending time getting associated with everything at the start of the doof. My group and I ventured back to the tent, as it was quite cold outside and it was bothering me. Everything was fine; we were tripping ridiculously (as expected) and having fun. I decided to take a bump of ketamine and clearly misjudged the amount on the spoon due to me tripping so hard, which was enough to send me into a K hole.

Roughly ten minutes later, things started to turn dark and signs of impending doom started to morph into my reality. Symbolisms of death and concerns that I had taken too many drugs started to plague my mind. Suddenly, my heart started racing uncontrollably and my throat started closing up. I started getting pains in my heart, liver, and lungs – all the signs and symptoms I knew which stated, "You have had a reaction or overdosed and your life is in danger."

At this stage I started to freak out a bit, calling out to my friends, telling them something is very wrong and that I needed help. But things were still morphing around me showing me I was about to die. In my panic I thought, "Keep your mind active and your body moving to fight it, you cannot die like this." So, I quickly walked outside the tent and vomited a bit. As I looked up I could tell there were people nearby but their faces were completely full of geometric patterns and colors. I couldn't make out details of who they were and I just said, "Sorry guys I am tripping out really hard," and started to walk in another direction.

As I walked, the whole world around me morphed into a completely different reality. Auditory hallucinations started clearly entering my spectrum of hearing, laughing at me and saying, "You brought this upon yourself," and, "You did it now." Everything in sight was red, black, and white, morphing so much that I knew I was in between the realm of the living and the dead. Something came to me and said, "If you never do drugs again we will let you live or if not you will die." I was battling them saying, "But I experience the Universe, myself and others through drugs. I do not see drugs as a bad thing; they help me on my quest of knowledge and truth in the Universe." They laughed and said, "Then if you cannot make the choice, we will make the choice for you." I felt my whole reality break apart.

I accepted my death and gave in to the Universe. I apologized to those I left behind in life and for dying the way I did, but at the same time that reality no longer existed, which gave me peace. I felt my consciousness break apart into fragments, as I heard what sounded like my voice going "Ahhhhhhhhh," fragmenting as if it had been digitally broken apart. As this was happening, I could feel every part of my soul breaking and fading into nothing – I was no longer Luke – Luke no longer existed. Complete ego death!

Suddenly in a void, I became distinctly aware of these other entities around me. The only way I can describe what they were or felt like is that they were the creators – high prestige royal entities without hierarchy. They knew and were everything. They were neither male nor female, but composed of the supreme consciousness. Higher vibrating entities that created me and my reality as a mere story to see how it would run – for amusement and fun (as the saying goes "Humans take seriously what the gods made for fun"). They praised the person I was in life and how they loved characteristics of my personality and what I did. They celebrated and laughed about all the funny and commendable things I had completed and the positive impact I had made on countless people along my lifetime.

I abruptly sunk deeper into the Universe, one with it, and my soul became one with this flowing machine of information. I was gliding through the Universe awaiting to be reborn into a new dimension or life. Shapes beyond the normal three dimensions were flying past me with the sounds and feeling of wind. As they flew past, I received information of the Universe so profound it is beyond human words or explanation – amazingly beautiful in both its simplicity and complexity. As this was all happening, I saw what seemed to be a civilization advanced far beyond humans in every sense of the word. You cannot imagine the power they possessed – there was no time, no space – it just was. I felt at one with them as I went through this system or machine.

Suddenly, the entities that created me came back and proceeded to say, "That story was great. Why don't we bring him back to see how it would have properly finished?" Right then, I felt a voting system between the countless numbers of creator entities take place. They voted "yes" to bring me back. All at once, parts of my consciousness and awareness started to form again. At this point I was nothing more than a singular atom endowed with consciousness, and from this single atom I proceeded to grow! They were restructuring me and my reality, reformatting everything back into existence. As they did, they were discussing whether to put me forward or back in life. "Should we grant him more finances or leave him where he was when he died? Should we take or leave certain parts of his personality and/or reality?" They were going back and forth, as I was put back together bit by bit. Then as I was nearly complete they granted me a gift. I started getting symbolism of the singularity, energy flowing through the Universe in an evident symbol of oneness. Then all of a sudden, I received this pure surge of energy and information. This was the information of the Universe – symbols of Buddha and the pine cone/pineal gland were clearly everywhere. At once, it was apparent what gift they had granted me, enlightenment through rebirth – I had become the true pure soul I was meant to be.

When reality was clear enough to function again, I found myself lying face down in the dirt a few tents away from my own. I struggled to get up and stumble back into the tent, while the entities were still making slight corrections to me and my reality. I remember yelling out to them to "Keep that!" as they were deciding whether to keep a trait of my personality or not. Once I was 100% back together, I gave them the 'perfect' symbol with my hand as if to commend them on putting me perfectly back together.

Once I was back, I took a Xanax and went straight to sleep. The whole experience took a huge toll and at the time all I wanted to do was sleep it off. This experience has profoundly changed me and my life for the better – forever. I am seeing my world as if I have a new set of eyes, everything is new and clear.

Clarity beyond perfection.

# RETURN TO THE TREE OF KNOWLEDGE

## Psilocybin

It was 7 p.m. on Christmas Eve. I was driving down the highway on my way to my best friend's apartment for something that had become quite important to me. I've had several past experiences with Psilocybin before but this was the one that would forever shift the very center of my being.

The routine was simple: brew the mushrooms into a tea. I had taken it with some ginger, since my stomach became easily upset. Then, under a dim light with a playlist of beautiful music, a notebook of questions, my best friend, and two sleeping pills that served as a sort of "abort" button should things get too hectic, I was prepared. I am not a doctor of any sort and while this procedure worked for me I would never advise anyone else do it.

As usual, my stomach was in knots. I am always a bit anxious going into these experiences. After all, this was the unmapped, virtually unexplored universe within as Terence McKenna called it. I drank, gathered up my blankets, a pillow, and settled in for another journey into the unknown.

Darkness. Fear. The sense of... leaving familiarity. Something many introverts are familiar with. Nothing too out of the ordinary yet. Then, a funny little thought. "This must be death. Or rather, a simulation of it." I looked up and asked my friend, "what do I do if it feels like I'm about to die?" She thought for a moment and said "I guess you should just go with it; die."

Blackness. Then… a light… a small hole of light peering through the darkness. I don't know if I walked to it or flew, but as I peered through this hole I felt myself suddenly begin to go into and through it and cross over into infinity. I could not believe what I was seeing or what I was feeling. Stars… planets… I was certainly not in my friend's apartment anymore. Floating amongst the celestial bodies I remained, until I ran into him.

He (or she) was of immense proportions. Stars for eyes, a galaxy for a body. I could not see where this deity ended or began, but his eyes, they had me. We did not speak, but I felt a sort of welcome in his presence. The deity proceeded to carry me through this vast universe until we reached a moon. One amongst many. It was the most beautiful sight I'd ever seen. In front of me was a moon about as big as a field, and on it were trees. Their bark was all white and only their leaves had color. But the leaves were of all colors constantly changing and glistening.

Upon setting foot on this elegant rock, I was flooded with a familiar feeling: home. Somehow, I'd been here before… many times. This. This place was my home. This place is where I had returned to time and time again. It is here that I spent my days until I was ready to grow more through the experience that can only be had on the other side; this side which we inhabited now. Suddenly, nothing seemed wrong. Everything had purpose. Life was worth living.

After a short while the deity appeared again. We locked eyes and I believe it knew that I had gotten what I was looking for: answers. Hope. A sign of things to come. So then, it was time to go, for it was not my time just yet. I was saddened. Had I been given a choice I would have remained, but I knew my work on Earth was not done yet. Off we went, past planets teeming with life and creatures with all too similar human tendencies. Past structures impossible to build in this reality. Pyramids of immense structure. This was the famed imaginatrix described by McKenna. By this point, I was shaken to my core and filled with awe. "This can't all be in my head. No way could I imagine all this off the bat. What am I to do now?"

Darkness. Color. Endless sky. A sea. The freeing of my imagination. The gift of creativity bestowed upon me. A thousand works of art unborn all flashed before my eyes at once. A reward for braving the unknown. Black again. Another small sliver of light. Onward and through. Then, I was back. I looked around. My friend and her cat had fallen asleep. 12 a.m. Christmas. My thoughts were silent. I was not sure how to process this.

To this day, I'm still not too certain about what happened, where I went, or what I saw. However, I know this. There is indeed a plan. A method to all this madness that haunts our world. And these chemicals, these mushrooms, they may hold the key to all the answers we've sought since we could question life. The journey is far from over. In fact, the journey may just never end, and I think I'd like that. Very much.

# HEART MEDICINE

## MDMA

My mother was 40 years old when she immigrated to the U.S. and met my father whom she married. The marriage was arranged by their families and even though they had never actually met before the wedding, they stayed together for nearly half a century until my dad passed way when he was 98 years old.

My mother had experienced many physical and emotional challenges in her life. She grew up in a small village and had to take care of farm animals and domestic needs in their family home. She was also abused by an alcoholic brother who would often beat her up, and one day even dragged her across the floor for not having prepared his dinner in time. During the Second World War, she was forced to witness the execution of her father and others by German Nazi soldiers as an example to the village of what would happen if anyone provided help to the U.S. military and its allies. After the war, she remained at home taking care of her invalid mother.

Many of the men that emigrated out of war torn Greece to other countries for better income and living opportunities continued to send money to their families back home. When he reached 50 years old, my father felt that he had paid his family obligations, including two wedding dowries for his sisters, and it was time for him to get married. He was matched with my mother and together they started a new life in Raleigh, North

Carolina where my father operated a small downtown diner.

Her uprooting from a little Greek village to a suburban life in a small southern city in the U.S. was challenging in many ways, but she assimilated as best as possible and was happy to not be living in the poverty and misery of her earlier life. She never learned enough English to be fully integrated in the community, but she made up for it by working hard at the restaurant and at home, as well as maintaining a beautiful flower and vegetable garden. Growing up for me was not only bilingual in language but also in culture. At the diner, my mother worked among typical Americans and cooked the standard Americana cuisine, but at home she kept her traditions active by speaking Greek, cooking Greek food, and being an active member of the local Greek Orthodox Church.

As happy as she was for her new life, my feelings as a child were that she was not allowing time to enjoy the aspects of the American dream as other families would. Work was a stringent duty and relaxation was not part of her program. As a child I wanted my parents to be more "American" and be active in "normal" activities such as bowling, picnics, baseball games, and drive-in movies. I remained puzzled as to why my parents never held hands, showed signs of affection or laughed like other people.

During my adolescent life in the 1960's, my mother felt threatened by my flourishing in the American culture that she never understood. The idea of me dating was equivalent to being a prostitute in her mind, as she believed couples should only be romantically together only in marriage. As I entered my psychedelic flowering, my mother was hysterical and felt terrified by my unconventional lifestyle, which she viewed as akin to worshiping demons. She even asked the local priest to do an exorcism on me because of my having a Jimi Hendrix poster on my bedroom wall.

As rough as it was for me growing up in a household where communications were not often very clear, I remained loyal in showing much affection and responsibility to my parents. Reciprocal displays of affection from them back to me were rare at best. One day I took my mother's hand and told her to touch my face and tell me she loved me. The more I tried pulling her hand to me, the more she resisted, to the point of screaming at me that she never knew love and would never be able to express it. Frail and almost 90 years old at the time, she started shaking and crying. I felt there were many experiences going on in her life affecting her emotions and it would be best if I backed out from any more pressuring her to show me the love that I asked for.

Along with my wife and our children, I moved back to Greece with my mother and lived with her for eight years. During that time, she rarely showed us any smiles or kind words. Her health deteriorated rapidly when she turned 99. She could no longer walk without trembling, nor do much in the way of independent action and thought. Her bitterness was more intense than ever and she made it clear that she wanted to die in her home and be buried with her ancestors. Her anger at us and the world in general continued to consume her passion.

It was on such an evening of her cursing my existence that

I reflected deeply on her situation. Under normal circumstances, I would find it unethical to give someone a drug without explaining to them the purpose and its possible side effects. But in this case of her being caught in such a web of emotional pain and negativity, I decided to give her the one dose of MDMA that I had been saving for a special occasion.

We were in her home, a traditional family home in a small agrarian Greek village. This was the ancestral house my mother had grown up in before immigrating to the United States as a young lady. The room she stayed in was exactly like she had left it fifty years prior, with the same bed and wall decorations.

As she grabbed the little white pill that I gave her, my mother hissed the question, "What are you giving me?" to which I replied that it was "heart medicine." Her retort was that I had been giving her poison to her heart all my life and here was one more intention of mine to kill her. I took a deep breath and felt the fear of a premonition that her experience could be a very very bad one. It would then be a decision that could haunt me for the rest of my life.

It turned out to be true. This decision has indeed had a significant impact on my life, but with a far better outcome than even I had anticipated. After giving her the "heart medicine" I said my good nights and left her alone.

Checking in half an hour later, I found her sitting on her bed gazing at an icon of the Virgin Mary. The fact that I saw her smiling was a hint that a profound event was manifesting. When I asked her how she felt, she softly said that "there were angels flying around the room." That was a trigger for me to run upstairs, wake up our son and tell him to come downstairs with his guitar – that we had important work to do with his grandmother.

For the next few hours we exchanged hugs with my mother and also shared her delight in listening to CDs of both Greek Orthodox religious hymns as well as her favorite Greek folk music. At times, my son would strum a few chords on his guitar while we sang about how much we loved her. When my wife came downstairs to be part of the miracle, she asked my mother how she was doing – to which my mom said in a very sweet tone, "this night will never end." My mother was no longer judgmental and mean. Her words, smiles, and touch were soft and loving. It was a blessing for all of us.

There was more amazement ahead. From that night on, for the last seven months of her life, my mother dropped her fear-based masking and let her heart express itself in a very beautiful way. No longer would she judge or criticize anyone, but instead say loving remarks. She would smile and ask to kiss us regularly every day. She no longer demanded I cut my beard, but asked if she could stroke it. She had previously refused to let her granddaughters take her to the village in her wheelchair – now she welcomed their brushing her hair, putting a flower in back of her ear, and taking her out for ice cream.

For most of her life she was carrying the impacted memories of abuse and trauma of her life that had become a centerpiece of her existence and how she viewed the world and others. Her devotion to religion focused more on Old Testament notions of guilt, shame, and sin rather than the relatively happier aspirations of the New Testament. Yet through all the heavy weight of such pain she carried, there was still a light within her waiting to find a way through the darkness.

What matters most is that one experience with the "heart medicine" brought lasting comfort in her remaining life and could well have helped her soul cross over more gently. The circle was more complete and her grandchildren will always remember her as being at peace with herself and the world. And of course, so will I.

# IT IS WHAT IT IS

## Salvia + DMT

Have you ever, in your however many years you've been exposed to this life, come into contact with something not human like you or I, or similar natured like the animals we pet and recycle? Something completely different that even the most experienced dimension dweller couldn't quite put their finger on?

The first time I met the machine elves, or should I say, elf, was the first time I properly broke through smoking DMT, and for those of you who are unfamiliar with the substance of DMT and this idea of "breaking through," I will try to break it down for you. When the right amount of DMT is administered, the user, without any warning, it's like a spaceship is diving through your mind, breaking through the walls of this dimension and catch a glimpse of an unknown dimension nestled deeply within the burrows of their own mind.

Mine sent me to a forest of some sort, where I was faced with a short ugly green figure with a pointy red hat. From the familiarity of fairy tales shown to me as a child, I knew what an elf looked like and here one was, standing right in front of me. This elf was a trickster; it didn't take a genius to point that out. He never took that smirky grin off his face, even when he spoke. The first time I met the elf, he had a reoccurring message for me: "It is what it is… it is what you make of it," he said over and over, shrugging and peering around. I could tell he was trying to make me understand something, if the reoccurring message wasn't enough.

Ever since that short but powerful DMT trip, those words have stuck with me like a magnet, often showing up everywhere around me, just those five words; "IT IS WHAT IT IS," friends' tattoos, written on bus seats, walls, advertisements, pretty much anywhere the elf could relay the message to me.

So, you think this is some pretty experimental shit to dab into? I haven't even gotten to the best part of this momentary mystery. Six months later, I decided to try smoking Salvia for the first time. Salvia Divinorum is an herbalist psychoactive plant whose effects are similar to that of DMT.

Before I smoked it around a circle of close friends in a tent in the wilderness, someone told me that Salvia is the kind of substance that requires the user to ask a certain question, and if that question has the intention of good, the spirits of the other dimension will greet you and answer your question. If unprepared, they would banish you from the dimension, never to return again.

I went into my first Salvia experience with an open mind and an open heart. What I wasn't expecting was the outcome. As I blew the smoke out, the trees began to wiggle and bend. I then noticed a shadow out of the corner of my eye. The shadow became clearer within seconds, and even I recognized this being. What gave up not his identity but his familiarity to me was the elf's voice as he ran laps around the tent, making it quite impossible to catch a glimpse of his structure, "You have seen me before, but you don't know my name…"

So "it is what it is." IT is what it is for a reason. Whether I see these five words somewhere, which will always bring me back to that experience, or if you see certain things that bring you back to a certain memory, whether it be a person, place or object, it is all subjective. This psychedelic experience taught me that everything is what it is for a reason. There is no point questioning it or fighting something that was always meant to be a certain way in the intrinsic flow of life. I realize, a year later, and now someone who has grown from this experience, that I was never meant to meet the elf personally, I was just meant to hear his message and apply it to my own life. I am getting the words tattooed on me this Sunday, as a constant reminder, which always will be.

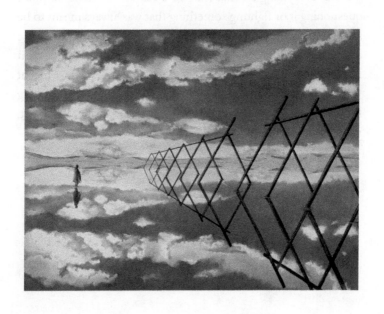

# SHOW ME THE TRUE NATURE OF THE UNIVERSE

## Ayahuasca

My cousin Zach and I were nervously rummaging around dimly lit rooms of our jungle bungalow, searching for the white cotton pants and tunics that we had bought in Iquitos to wear to ceremony. The sun had set and day had already given way to night. We put on our robes in the soft glow of a single light bulb hanging from the low ceiling. The soft hum of the distant generator assured us that there would be several more minutes of power.

Night in the Amazon was unlike any other. The lack of nearby cities or villages fostered a more complete darkness that was only punctuated by the lights suspended in the cosmos. It was obvious that the candles we had been given would not burn through the whole night, a thought that only added to my anxiety of what the night had in store.

The light may have died, but the jungle had sprung to life. Songs from hordes of insects and armies of frogs desperately calling out for mates created an almost deafening symphony in the darkness. Our eyes had no way of knowing it, but it was clear that we were far from alone in the rainforest. It was a reassuring revelation, but also one that was simultaneously, equally disconcerting.

The soft glow of the light only enhanced the bioluminescence given off by our white clothes. Cole had explained to us that white clothes would help protect from dark energy and allow light energy to more fully flow through us. I was initially skeptical at this claim and was reluctant to spend one hundred soles on clothes that would never be worn again. White has never been my color.

We were quiet, taking turns playing the cheap nylon string guitar Zach had bought only minutes before getting on the boat to Altiplano. Zach's fingers danced along the fret board, picking out several songs including Eric Clapton's *Tears in Heaven*. Every so often we would exchange quiet, nervous looks, almost as if telepathically reading each other's unease as the clock neared 7:30 p.m. Finally, we heard talking in the distance, followed by a bouncing light and the sound of rubber boots crossing the small wooden bridge by our bungalow.

"Ceremonia," beckoned a soft voice outside the bug-netted door. The voice belonged to one of the Guardians, a member of Altiplano's staff whose job it was to escort us to and from ceremony each night. Our instructions had urged us to bring our pillows, a blanket, water, and a headlamp with us. With full arms, we slipped into our rubber boots and quietly followed the Guardian over the wet, root-ridden jungle floor.

Once across the bridge, we let out gasps of awe as we got our first glimpse of the Amazonian night sky. Headlamps were extinguished and thousands, if not tens of thousands, of stars and other celestial bodies crowded the vast darkness of the cosmos. "Fucking rad," I said incredulously as I craned my neck to investigate the foreignness of the southern hemisphere's vision of space in the summer. I had never seen the Milky Way so distinctly. A muttered word from the Guardian urged us to continue.

We clumsily stomped up the wooden stairs to the maloca, depositing tracks of mud on the first several steps. In the dim candle light, we could see Fabian was already seated at a mat on the far side of the room, nearest to the bathroom. Zach and I said quiet 'hellos' but the conversation stopped there as we each chose the next mats in line and made ourselves comfortable.

Looking around the large circular room I noticed the table at the front where two lit candles sat next to an unfamiliar two-pronged string instrument and a bottle of Agua de Florida, a fragrant tincture made from distilled flower petals. To the table's left there was a short hall to a bathroom with three toilets, surely there for us to use if our purging took the form of diarrhea. The thought of finding that bathroom in the dark while under the influence of the Medicine was intimidating and made me quietly hope that I would just have to vomit instead. Next to each mat was a small plastic bucket for vomitus. Luckily Altiplano didn't serve dinner on ceremony days, otherwise the bucket may have been too small to contain the contents of our rice and lentil laden stomachs.

The rest of the group slowly started to filter in, led by the other Guardians. Shayne took the mat next to me and Kim took the one beside his so all four of us would be close during the ceremony. More nervous glances were exchanged along with jokes about how we all looked as if we were about to be baptized again.

Our translator Arienne entered with Jose and another elderly man with a small frame and a soft, contented expression on his weathered face, who I assumed to be Horatio. Jose procured a tall glass bottle of a dark liquid and set it on the front table before finding the center of the room and lighting a third candle.

Conversation ceased and Arienne gave a welcome to us on behalf of the two curanderos. She said that tonight would be a very special ceremony and expressed Jose's hopes for the forest spirits to be with us in ceremony to protect and look over us. We were reminded that the newcomers would be receiving a smaller, introductory dose of Ayahuasca in order for the Medicine to establish a relationship with each of our unique bodies. It was also to serve the purpose of a diagnostic assessment of how we respond to the Medicine to inform our later doses. Jose reassured us to have trust and patience, telling us that he had thirty years of experience and that Horatio was going on fifty years participating in ceremony.

"Ayahuasca is a powerful medicine, capable of healing many ailments," he said in Spanish with a quiet confidence. "The Icaros that you will hear tonight are to guide the spirits and each of you in your journey. Some will be sung in Spanish and others in native Quechua. Now, let us begin."

We all watched as he uncorked the glass bottle and put his mouth to the opening and begin rhythmically blowing into the neck, making low whistles. After a moment, the bottle was passed to Horatio who proceeded to do the same. Then they each took turns pouring Ayahuasca into a small cup and tilting their heads back, reaching for a cup of water. Jose then beckoned for Fabian to sit at his side. Fabian slowly rose to his feet before nervously walking over to the table. Jose poured a small amount in the same cup and blew into the cup's contents, blessing it, before passing it to Fabian, who hesitated a moment before knocking the cup back. Zach then followed suit.

I was already on my feet and on my way to the table as Zach returned to his mat. I sat next to Jose, embraced by the light of the candles, as he put a gentle hand on my back and smiled with a loving softness that spoke to the unmistakable wisdom behind his eyes. He blessed the cup once more and passed it to me. It was about a quarter full, and by the light of the candle, I could see darker specks in the dark red liquid. I closed my eyes and raised the cup to my lips; the thick liquid went down quickly but left a complex, pungent taste in my mouth. It was kind of sweet, kind of spicy, and kind of savory, and in light of the bland food I had been eating for the past several days, I was grateful for its robust flavor.

As I walked back to my mat, the realization truly dawned on me that there was no turning back now. The familiar phrase "Ride the lightning" once again crossed my mind and I sat cross-legged, smoking a mapacho, and internally re-enforcing my intention for the evening as the rest of the group received their doses.

After the administration of the Ayahuasca, the curanderos began at opposite sides of the rooms, taking the Agua de Florida to rhythmically blow it gently onto each of our hands and use it to mark small crosses on our hearts and foreheads. Jose then took his lit mapacho, a rolled cigarette with jungle tobacco, and proceeded to form a smoke circle around the group to provide additional protection from malevolent spirits. Upon completion of the smoke ring, Jose returned to sit at the front of the room as we all basked silently in the light of the candles waiting for the Medicine to take effect. Several more silent minutes passed before Jose grabbed a leaf fan and rose to extinguish each of the three candles, and we were plunged into darkness.

I heard the leathery fluttering of a bat fly through the un-netted windows of the maloca and whiz past my ear in the darkness, and to my surprise I didn't jump but remained focused on my intention. "Show me the true nature of the Universe," I repeated quietly in the confines of my mind.

Jose began singing. His voice was ethereal in its tone, "Medicina poderoso, Ayahuasca..." I began picking out as many lines as I could, sometimes struggling to translate as the tune and rhythm of the singing disrupted the usual pattern of how the words are spoken in conversation. "Powerful medicine, Ayahuasca. Protect us tonight. Doctor plant, chacurnita." The tune was heavy with smooth and drawn out legatos across large sweeps of notes, while the words were obviously part of a carefully orchestrated mantra. Despite the predetermined words, the influence of the Ayahuasca informed the curanderos how to sing the Icaros with each unique ceremony.

Someone to my left puked abruptly, but Jose's voice did not falter. More gut-wrenching vomiting soon followed affirming that Fabian's purging had begun.

I started to feel my heart beat stronger throughout my body; it became a pulsation that felt as though my heart was pumping the thick Ayahuasca through my blood vessels, away from my heart to penetrate the extremities of my body. My body began to slowly rock back and forth with the pulses, as if to embrace the sensation. An unmistakable sense that every component of my body was being looked at, analyzed by the Ayahuasca as it intuitively began assessing my very being. It was as if I was being scanned, finding points of strength and weakness within myself that even I was even not consciously aware of. The feeling was one of unprecedented intimacy and a level of comprehensive understanding that I had no idea was possible.

Clouds must have gathered above the maloca as a soft rain began to fall on the thatched palm roof, the pitter patter providing a background of static to Jose's singing. The small gaps between the woven fronds allowed for microscopic droplets to fall in a cool, almost imperceptible vapor upon my outstretched body.

As the assessment continued to inspect my body, I laid down on my mat. My eyes were closed but pinpricks of twinkling light started to appear directly above me in the dark field that occupied my mind. My body became overwhelmed by a tingling vibration that slowly grew in intensity as my field of vision opened up to become a starry night sky before my very eyes. The tingling spread to all of my body, with the exception of the right half of my head and face, until it reached a frequency that seemed to harmoniously meld with that of the rest of the matter in my environment. It was a glorious sensation of letting go of my physical body through full assimilation into my surroundings. However, the disparity of sensation between the right side of my head and the rest of my body allowed me an avenue through which I could still ground myself in my physical body.

The rain had now begun to fall heavier and more intensely, growing into a healthy jungle shower that seemed to create a comforting barrier around the maloca. Beside me, more violent puking erupted from both Zach and Fabian. Although conscious of the purging going on around me, my eyes remained closed and I continued to focus on maintaining an even rhythm to my breath. I was so relaxed that sometimes my transitions from inhale to exhale were almost imperceptible.

The sky that I saw open up above me was changing. Spectacular forms of monolithic scale that looked as though they were hewn from technological crystals took shape in a new celestial dimension. I was moving, soaring through some atmosphere populated by wispy, white clouds and these mysterious suspended structures of deep azure and radiant gold. Hurtling on, I saw that not only were there more of these structures, but that some of them were slowly changing and taking on new shapes.

Suddenly, I found myself in the presence of a vast new form. A seemingly boundless mechanical device comprised of an incalculable number of interconnected gold components: gears, arms, springs, levers, dials, columns of interlocking pieces moving tirelessly. The Universe. But it was made clear that this device was a metaphor for the sake of my incredibly small realm of experience to make sense of an entity that is vastly beyond my comprehension.

I continued to float within the mechanical behemoth, taking note of the columns of interlocking pieces that bore a resemblance to combination locks or the tumblers in a safe. Each column was a stack of cells with individual organisms that spun and rotated in tandem with the others around it. The overwhelming sense that the Universe was just as much a puzzle solving apparatus as it was a cosmic clock pervaded my mind. Not only that, but it was a living system with nothing at the helm. Each and every one of the magnificent parts of the behemoth all played a particular role in governing how the machine functioned, and did so eternally.

This system was entirely self-sufficient; creating an infinite number of puzzles for itself as it simultaneously created an infinite number of solutions. The puzzles were characterized by constraints of limited amounts of matter and finite amounts of energy, while the solutions were involved with finding ways for energy and matter to come together in a harmonious equilibrium that was healthy for maintaining the system.

Having all of these puzzles and solutions could have looked like the omniscience of "God" that I had been told of many times, but this consciousness was far more beautiful and just shy of perfect. The beautiful imperfection of this consciousness came from knowing the puzzles and the solutions, but not always knowing the circumstances of when, where, and with exactly what components brought about the harmony that the Universe so desperately tried to cultivate. Experience through trial and error is the key to the eternal expansion of this collective consciousness, each life playing a vital role in providing another piece to the grand puzzle. All matter has a life, whether it is in the form of an igneous rock, a blade of grass, or in the form of a human being and each and every one of them are a body of experience in the eyes of the Universe; energy acting upon a body of matter as a test of what can be created given circumstantial constraints.

Given the imperfect consciousness of the Universe, there will inevitably be successes but there will also be failures. But there is no need for despair. Even the "failures" are necessary for the path towards creating a more perfect consciousness; just as much is learned from failing as is learned from success, and there are rarely instances that demand a balance is found on the first attempt. And if at first you don't succeed, try, try again. Eventually the Universe will find equilibrium.

The interconnectedness of all things had never been made as clear to me as it did when I was in the presence of such an awe-inspiring entity. It inspired a humbling gratitude to sweep over my being, as I realized the need for me to acknowledge how indebted I was to all the things that came before me and all the things that would come after me. The Universe depends on us all. Consciousness is "God," a term that seems incredibly inadequate at describing what I was witnessing. "God" is found within in each of us in the form of consciousness, and each consciousness is a part of the collective consciousness of the Universe. As products of the Universe, we are not only individually whole, but also part of an infinite whole.

As quickly as the mechanical Universe had appeared, it dissipated into black.

What faded into view next was a vibrant picture of two pairs of hands, one male and one female, connecting over a red

126

and white flower mandala on a patch of grass. The field of vision only extended as far as the mid forearms and there was no other anatomical information to confirm the identities of the figures. Not that I needed it.

I knew that these were my girlfriend Caitlin's and my hands. Our fingers interlocked and our palms took turns enfolding the other's in an intimate moment of exploration of each other. I could feel that I was physically smiling and soon a new, yet very similar pair of hands took Caitlin's and my place.

Once again there were no additional visual signifiers of identity, but I knew they belonged to my friends Nikki and Jeff. There was no mandala. They were holding each other's hands over a table which I knew was located in the bar that I worked at. I was perplexed at why I was being shown someone else's relationship, but settled that it must just be affirming the legitimacy of their affections for each other. Upon reaching this sufficient realization, I thought of my other friends who were in relationships. I tried to picture Travis' and Meagan's hands in a similar manner, but was surprisingly denied any inkling of that image.

In the space that followed, out of the darkness came a vision of the white ceremonial clothes that I was wearing being consumed by fire. Although the specific reason for this was not clear, what was clear was that these clothes were destined to be an offering; an effigy that was to be destroyed by flame.

The visions then started to dull, and almost as a parting farewell, the Universe consolidated itself into the facsimile of a cosmic face and winked at me. It seemed surprisingly cheeky, but it was an unmistakable message that said, "Here's a glimpse, but this is far from everything there is."

I opened my eyes to find that Jose had re-lit the candle in the middle of the room. I slowly sat up in awe of what I had just been taught, the flickering flame of the candle bringing me back into existing in my body, conscious of the room full of awakening dreamers. To my left, Zach was smoking a cigarette and turned to look at me with wide eyes of bewilderment that left me with a burning curiosity of what he had experienced.

Jose spoke and Arienne translated, "That concludes our ceremony tonight. Feel free to stay in the maloca as long as you want, the Guardians will be here to take you home when you are ready."

Everyone remained sitting on their mats. Cole and Andy exchanged a few indiscernible words across the room, but we largely remained silent. Objects still left tracers as they moved through my field of vision, almost creating the sense that I was witnessing objects in multiple planes separated by minute intervals in space. Elation was the only word adequate enough to describe my state of being. My intention had been entirely fulfilled; I had seen what most people would describe as "God."

After a few minutes, Zach and I gathered our pillows and water bottles and found our muddy boots. One of the Guardians led us down the steps. Our feet clumsily found each step as we struggled to maintain our balance. Once in the clearing, we noticed that the rain clouds had dispersed and were met by an even more impressive view of the cosmos, almost as if Ayahuasca granted us the capacity to gaze deeper into its vastness. We stood in awe for a few moments before continuing on to our bungalow. At the door we bid goodnight to the Guardian and thanked him for his help.

Zach and I didn't talk much following the ceremony, and I generated most of the meager dialogue in the candlelight. From my seat in the hammock, I could see Zach slowly smoking a mapacho, his face indicating an internal grappling with whatever he just saw.

We went to bed early that night. The jungle must have been merciful to us as I don't recall being kept up with a barrage of mysterious rustlings among the leaves. Instead, I was sung to sleep by the lullaby of the chorus of frogs, birds, and bugs.

The next morning, I awoke early to the sound of another rain shower and a bowl of freshly cut pineapple, watermelon, papaya, and banana that had been delivered to our bungalow an hour before. My body showed no sign of the mental or physical exhaustion that often followed my mushroom trips. What seemed to be taking its place was a clarity, humility, and gratitude for the awe-inspiring experience of the night before and the incredible natural world that provided me such an opportunity.

Zach was still sleeping deeply as I put on my boots and began walking to the dining hall for breakfast, eager to hear about everyone's journeys.

I sat at the table, joining Andy, Shayne, and Kim who were talking quietly and intermittently with one another. We exchanged 'good mornings' and they asked how I felt. I reported that I felt very well, and still elated. Our conversation then turned to how incredibly intense the Ayahuasca experience was, all expressing some anxiety and excitement as to what we would be in store for tonight with full doses of the Medicine.

We ate a breakfast of eggs, fried bananas, fruit juice, and a bowl of soup consisting of a bland broth with some cabbage and carrots floating just below its surface. Our conversation didn't delve into the particulars of our individual experiences, as we focused mainly on replenishing our energy.

Shortly after our meal, we were joined by Zach and Cole. Cole wore a look of zeal that reflected his eagerness for our next ceremony, hopeful to once more expand his understanding of his calling as a healer. On the other hand, Zach's face wore the same look of bewilderment that I had seen after last night's ceremony.

As Shayne, Zach, and I sat at one of the long wooden tables, we inquired about Zach's well-being. He seemed to silently ponder for a moment before answering. Slowly, in a low, purposeful tone, he told us that in Cusco, the curandero Augustine had made a shocking prophecy in a coca leaf reading about Zach's trek to the jungle and that Augustine's prophecy had already come to fruition in the first ceremony. This came as a surprise to us all. Many of us that had been given coca leaf readings went into them with a healthy skepticism of the clairvoyant abilities of such practices and Zach may have been the most skeptical of the group.

Cole and Andy soon joined our table, and Shayne encouraged his brother to share his experience with them. Upon the second recount, their faces showed the same surprise that Shayne and mine did. Our conversation then took a turn towards the healing powers that Ayahuasca had on those who came seeking liberation from substance abuse and addiction, focusing on how it changes one's inner dialogue and self-definition in relation to their past. As usual, Andy's comments were largely based on the words of famous yogis. As wise as these words may have been, in our present company and with Andy's lack of personal experience with addiction, his comments were somewhat insensitive. The rest of us were quick to try and direct the conversation and comments in a more constructive and thoughtful trajectory and began to discuss the power of "I" statements.

This was a topic that I had thought about a great deal several years earlier when I had really begun to refine the maturing, young adult that I was to become. "I" statements are the most powerful declarations that an individual can make in terms of their self-definition, a constant act of empowerment and awareness of one's Self.

We talked about how the translation of "God" in the Bible equates with "I am," perhaps the two most powerful words that can be conceived by the human mind. So much of our internal dialogue can be influenced by these two words, both in ways that empower us, as well as relinquish power over our being. I was eager to share my philosophy of our inherent nature as "gods," beings capable of all the divine powers that the main religions attribute to a supreme being of God. There were several nods when I stated that all of us are capable of creating and taking life, being creators and destroyers of worlds, the privilege of accumulating a seemingly infinite amount of knowledge, and ultimately being the writers of our own lives and destinies. I relished in the validation that I received from these wise men that I respected, all of them almost a decade older than I was. It was a validation that made me immediately grow closer to them, seeing us as a group of friends and brothers. In conclusion, we all acknowledged the need for us to implement this divine right of self-definition in our conversations with Ayahuasca, using it to give us both strength and guidance as we confronted our truest selves. Our conversation dwindled down until we parted ways, some of us to nap while others either read or played card games.

One by one, we each had an opportunity to speak with Jose about our experiences and let him further assess how we uniquely interact with the Medicine. I was particularly eager to share with him my thoughts and feelings.

When my time came, Arienne found me in the dining hall and beckoned me to the lounge area. I followed her, both of us making gentle thuds as our feet rose and fell on the weathered, wooden planks. We sat on couches adorned with the Chipibo fabric that we were now so familiar with. Jose was sitting with his soft and peaceful demeanor and eventually spoke asking if I needed Arienne to translate. I replied in Spanish that I knew a good amount of Spanish but would prefer to have a translation to ensure that I didn't miss anything that he had to say. He gave an understanding nod and said "Bueno. How was your experience with the Ayahuasca? How did you feel?"

I began to recount that it had been a very gentle experience that gave me a great deal of information that I had hoped to attain that night. He seemed to know that I hadn't needed to purge, as he commented on how calm I had looked throughout ceremony. A smile of deep satisfaction spread across his gentle face as I told him that the Universe had coyly winked at me and he reaffirmed that there would be much more to learn. We sat smiling for a moment before he reminded me that there would be a floral bath in several hours. I thanked him for his time and reinforced my excitement for our next ceremony.

As the jungle air finally began to cool and four o'clock got near, Zach and I put on our swim trunks, gathered our towels and made the hike to meet for the flower baths. We walked across the hard clay ground in our boots, trying our best to avoid tromping on the swaths of leaf-cutter ants that were creating highways in the grass.

After a short walk, we came to the sauna building which lay on the swampy edge of the river. A few dozen tree trunks shot up through the cool, murky water to form a canopy above us, the last strong beams of afternoon sun poking through gaps in the foliage. Jose was standing outside the sauna with several large, plastic tubs of water next to him. It became clear that this bath was not going to be one where we each lounged, almost submerged in warm, floral water. The buckets of clear river water were full of leafy, green clippings of various flowers and herbs from the refugio's garden that Jose had picked earlier in the day. We stood next to each other in our swimwear; everyone had come with the exception of Shayne and Kim, and awaited our turns to be bathed.

Baptized may be a better word for it. One by one we stood in front of Jose and Kelly as they filled buckets with the fragrant water and tossed it over us. I laughed as each of the Canadians flinched and squealed at the frigid water, finding their reaction ironic. We were encouraged to refrain from brushing the clippings off our bodies, allowing it to cleanse and permeate our skin. However, they granted us permission to get any uncomfortable bits that the rush of the water had forced down our swim trunks, which we were all grateful. The Earthy aroma of the concoction was indeed refreshing and seemed to at least mask the sweaty musk that we were surely accumulating from the jungle climate. Our bodies dried and we slowly shed bits of green as we walked back to our bungalows.

Several hours passed and once again the sun began to set on the Amazon jungle in a brilliant palette of oranges, reds, and violets. Shayne and Kim had come by to visit Zach and I at our bungalow before we headed to our second ceremony. We conversed for a while under the light of our lantern powered by a distant generator that hummed aggressively off in the distance, a sound that seemed strikingly out of place among the incessant calls of the nocturnal jungle.

Zach and I were disappointed to find out that Kim would once again not be partaking in the Medicine in that night's ceremony. As Shayne and Kim prepared to return to their own bungalow in preparation for ceremony, we each gave Kim a hug of encouragement and told her we loved her. Once out of the bug netted door, their voices and light of their headlamps faded into the darkness.

Several minutes passed as Zach and I once again put on our white ceremonial clothes. We sat listening to the chorus of awakening bugs and frogs. My excitement to learn something new and profound largely drowned out the nervousness that had plagued me the night before. In the dim light, it was hard to tell if Zach shared my excitement or was bracing himself for another harrowing night as he smoked several mapacho.

All of a sudden, our heads swiveled almost in unison as we heard a jarring sound from just outside the walls of our bungalow. It was a loud, breathy, almost speech-like sound that stood out amongst the usual rustling foliage. We didn't know what we expected to find. The lime green bug netting that formed the walls just barely obfuscated the world that lay just outside of them. Our gazes lingered on what we could not see for a moment before we looked uneasily at each other, both of us slightly unnerved. After a couple more drags of Zach's mapacho, we heard it again.

Whatever was making the bizarre sound seemed to have shifted several feet before producing the eerie sound. Even with all my substantial knowledge of rainforest animals, I was utterly perplexed at what kind of creature could make such a sound. It sounded like nothing I had heard before, and it sounded almost supernatural and caused the hairs on my arms and neck to stand on end. In my discomfort I joined Zach in nervously smoking another mapacho as we looked at each other. Silently, we exchanged looks that displayed how freaked out we both were. Two grown men sitting scared in the jungle like two young kids camping after hearing a particularly scary ghost story.

Zach nervously rose from his wooden seat and walked to the bathroom. I could faintly hear the sound of urine hitting porcelain, before the sound returned again, louder and even closer to discernible words than before. And it was just outside the bathroom. Almost immediately, I heard Zach call from the bathroom, "What did you say?" I was scared before, but I was now terrified. It was clear that Zach had thought this last vocalization, for lack of a more fitting word, had been me talking to him. As he came back from the bathroom, he must have seen my terror even before I muttered that I hadn't said anything.

The ominous presence outside our bungalow was now utterly undeniable and making itself absolutely known. We both picked up headlamps and walked to the limits of the bug netting, shining the beams through the tiny holes into the darkness. The lamps were only capable of illuminating a short range outside and failed to expose the source of the sounds. Unsatisfied and perplexed by the lack our lack of findings, we returned to our seats huddled at the center of the room, struggling to rationalize our fear of this invisible tormentor.

As several more minutes passed spent smoking and trying to quell our disquieted composures, we heard boot steps on the dense, clay of the path leading to our bungalow and a loud spitting of our Guardian coming to take us to ceremony. In my head I was scared for him as he neared the spot where we believed the presence to be hiding and briefly considered calling out to warn him, but then realized how infantile I would seem to a man who lived in and knew the jungle far better than I did.

We proceeded to follow him nervously into the clearing. Dense clouds produced by the dense jungle hung above us, blocking the magnificent view of the cosmos that we had seen blocking the magnificent view of the cosmos that we had seen the night before.

Our bungalow was the closest to the maloca and once again we were among the first to arrive for ceremony. I sat cross-legged and proceeded to calm my mind and push the thought of the voice we had heard out of my mind. As the others began to filter in and assume the mats they had occupied the night before, I focused on formulating and refining my intention for the evening. I had learned about the vastness of the Universe, but now I wanted to learn about bettering my Self. I took a great deal of care searching for the right words to define my desire to learn, ultimately settling on "Please send me my spirit animal to teach me to become my higher Self."

Once again, the participants of the ceremony began to filter into the maloca. My cousins and friends were always noticeable, even from across the room in the dim candle light, appearing in the doorway looking like shimmery specters in their white ceremony clothes. Jose and Horatio arrived with Arienne and the tall, glass bottle of dark Ayahuasca.

There was a good deal of shuffling about as everyone made themselves comfortable, ensuring that buckets, water bottles, mapacho, and lighters were all within a familiar arm's reach when the candles were snuffed out. The thrum of the generator could still be heard in the distance.

After repeating my intention several more times, I opened my eyes to the room and began watching Jose prepare his materials. Horatio was sitting several feet to Jose's left, craning his neck to look at something near the entrance of the maloca. I could not see the expression worn on his aged face in the candlelight, but his stare lingered, unmoving for several moments.

Thinking we may be waiting on another person, I took a mental roll call of the room. Fabian. Zach. Me. Shayne. Kim. Curtis. Danielle. Kelly. Andy. Cole. Chris. Everyone was present for ceremony. It couldn't be that Horatio was looking for someone.

He then turned to Jose and muttered something in Spanish that I was unable to make out. Jose then peered into the same patch of darkness that Horatio had, and there his gaze also lingered. It seemed as though the curanderos were aware of something that the rest of us were oblivious to, something that demanded their attention, delaying the ceremony for a few moments. I was struggling to retain the calmness that I had finally regained after the disconcerting experience we had in our bungalow. The ominous feeling of a presence which I could not see returned.

The shaman eventually exchanged a few soft words and redirected their attention to the beings within the room. Whatever it was that had drawn their gaze seemed to not be of immediate importance, and that gave me a small sense of relief.

"Tonight we will begin our healings," Arienne began translating for Jose. "Each night we will work personally with three of you. Tonight we will be healing Fabian, Kim, and Chris." Jose pointed a beam at each one to indicate to Horatio where each was sitting so they could more easily find them later in the darkness.

The shaman sanctified the Medicine, drank, and one by

one, we each rose to partake. This time we were each given our full potency dose. We then sat again in silence, basking in the candlelight while it lasted.

After several minutes, Jose stood and walked to the middle of the room. With one swoop of the leaf fan, both the candle and distant power generator went out. It was an eerie, unplanned orchestration that made the plunge into complete darkness seems even more austere.

I lied on my back, my head cradled in the cushion of my pillow. My eyes shut and I began focusing on the filling and emptying of my lungs with the fresh jungle air. Soon Jose's voice began singing the familiar Icaro from the night before, only this time with a slightly different melody. I was eager for the same geometric patterns to manifest in the field of my mind, dancing to the smooth legatos of Jose's singing. My body anticipated the warm, vibrating sensation to take hold of me and sweep me out of the physical room. I waited for what felt like an hour, with only the faint inklings of the Medicine taking effect.

Earlier at lunch, Kelly had told us that if you felt the desire to go deeper or that you needed a larger dose at any point in the ceremony, you could ask for it and it would be given to you. My impatience mounted until I got up the guts to rise to my feet, and slowly make my way to the table.

Horatio had taken over the singing of the Icaros and as Jose sensed me approaching the table, he shone a dim light to help me wend my way in the darkness. I sat on his right side as he put a fatherly hand on my shoulder. "Mas?" he questioned me. "Si, por favor. No siento mucho." He found the small cup that we each drank from, filled it again halfway with Ayahuasca, and blessed it before handing it to me. I tilted my head back and swallowed. The Medicine was slowly beginning to taste more and more acrid with each dose, and I made a sour face as I handed the cup back to Jose. With a series of slightly unsure steps, I found my mat with the help of Jose's light. Surely this would be sufficient for me to learn another profound lesson.

Waiting in the darkness, my impatience continued to mount. I was sitting with eager eyes opened and my legs crossed, trying to keep my back as straight and strong as I had seen Cole's and Andy's in yoga practice.

Just then another soft light appeared and I saw Andy make the same trek to the front of the room to get a second helping. I was perplexed. We had been told that this was a particularly strong batch of medicine and that it wouldn't take much to elicit strong visions. Two of us had now gone up for more. Was this a different batch than the night before?

I was growing more and more frustrated. A feeling of being forsaken by God started to take over me, as I was reminded of the story of Jesus' suffering in Gethsemane. I had witnessed the nature of the Universe and had been taught so much last night, but that could not possibly be all I was meant to learn in the jungle. I was surrounded by my family, friends, and several strangers, yet I felt utterly alone, left behind to fruitlessly wait as they all took a journey into the realm of wisdom and knowledge. It was as if anger was about to begin surging through my veins, like I had felt the Ayahuasca do the night before.

I could hear the guttural heaving as several of my

companions begin to purge violently into their buckets. As I sat in the darkness, my mind was beginning to concoct vivid images fueled by my mounting frustration and loneliness.

The first consisted of a tiny orb of white light giving off a dim, yet illuminating aura. The orb was in a disorienting space, void of solid forms or any sense of horizon or grounding. As the orb hung in the air, a dense, abyssal darkness was condensing around it. It plumed as tendrils of blackness emerged from the shroud as if to further close in on the orb and slowly suffocate it. Both of these entities were very much animated, personified as if they were participants suspended in a display of predator and prey. The darkness swirled with an inky fluidity around the orb, searching for a hole in the aura that emanated from the orb's core, but was foiled at each attempt. Despite its infinitesimal size, the body of light remained undiminished by the vast darkness which beset it. My eyes were open at this point and as this image permeated my mind, I struggled to determine whether I had truly begun my conversation with Ayahuasca yet.

As the image of the orb faded, it was replaced by a one of an immensely foggy waterfront. Whether I was seeing a freshwater or marine shore was unclear; the water and thick, misty atmosphere blended together beautifully in a wash of silver-grey. The scene reminded me of the serene, Japanese ink scenes of sublime tranquility in nature that I had seen in museums. A dark wooden dock jutted out of the fog and over the glassy, undisturbed water providing the only sense of physicality to the scene. At the end of the dock was a young man. Dressed in a drab, grey tunic and matching pants, he was

141

kneeling penitently with hands pressed together, but his meditation was interrupted by the slumping of his body as it fell almost lifelessly towards the water. The image was frozen, leaving me with a disquieting anxiety as I helplessly witnessed this young man head towards what seemed like a watery fate. His body just hung there, never nearing the water's surface.

Suddenly, I was free of the young man and his impending fate. But relief was not what followed in their wake. A choppy sea of darkness pressed itself to the forefront of my mind. The dark waves crested and met a dark sky void of many starry pinpricks of light, a dense blackness hanging low overhead. A small origami boat rode the disturbed waters. Flames began to consume its papery sail and hull with tongue-like lapping, illuminating the scene with a gut-wrenching orange glow. The consistent theme of violently disrupted tranquility was unnerving and demanded that I work to keep a calm composure.

Once more, the image dissolved. This time I saw a familiar scene resembling the layout of the maloca that I was sitting in. It was dark, but a single candle burned in the center. There was a semi-circle of mats, pillows, and blankets around the blanket all showing signs of disarray as they had all been occupied and vacated. All of them but one. Another young man was still sitting on one of the mats that was just left of the middle of the arc. He was alone and embodied my feelings of forsakenness as his companions had embarked on a journey and left him to wait nervously by the light of the candle.

As I continued to brace myself for the incredible sensations I had experienced the night before, I was still skeptical that the Medicine was really taking full effect. So in a desperate last attempt, I once again rose to my feet. This time my steps fumbled as they crossed the wooden floor, hoping not to find themselves landing on a hairy tarantula. Jose once again guided me to the table but this time greeted me with a soft face displaying a healthy dose of confusion. Or perhaps it was concern; either way, I'm sure it mirrored the expression I wore on my own face.

"Todovia no siento nada," I told him, explaining that I was still struggling to be plunged into the Medicine. He filled the ceramic cup again two-thirds full blessed it, and passed it to me to partake.

I sat again for a few minutes, free of the dark images that occupied my mind. My frustration and impatience were at their peak, but with a final dose I was also hopeful that something would happen. "Please let me learn something tonight," I thought to myself, almost offering up an open invitation to the Universe. "Anything."

My stomach gave a small gurgle as I began to contemplate that perhaps tonight I was meant to learn from just being present in the room, holding space for others, and enjoying being in the jungle air, listening to its song.

The shaman had begun their healings. Both worked with Fabian, their joint abilities seeming to draw out even more violent purging than before. Then it was Kim's turn.

I was laying down listening to the Icaros helping cleanse Kim, finally having reached a peace with my night, gazing through the windows of the maloca when it happened.

It was though I had been struck, so suddenly seized by

something dark, powerful, and ominous. I could not see my attacker with my eyes, nor feel it with my tactile senses, but it hit hard and fast, shaking me to my soul. My whole body went cold, sweat starting to pour from my forehead as it started to quake.

Then came the smell.

It was a pungent odor, one that seemed to engulf my whole being; one that reeked of death and shit. I was now quaking and experiencing blackouts, losing connection with my corporeal body as my attacker began to fill it with darkness. Utterly disoriented, I thought perhaps I had shit myself in one of the lapses in my consciousness. I quickly stood up on my mat to check for any sign of incontinence, only to find none. After only a couple seconds on my feet, weakness drew me back down. I was now feeling absolutely helpless at the hands of my assailant, and losing connection with my body quickly.

"Ayuda," I called out seeking help in feebly spoken Spanish, while also trying not to alarm the others in their vulnerable state. After calling out, I became terrified at the prospect of the shaman not knowing that I was calling out to them, and the possibility of them dismissing my calling out as addressing something in a vision I might be having.

After another brief blackout, I gained enough strength to call out again, more loudly and desperate this time. "Ayudame." I called out into the darkness, hopefully loud enough to be heard over the Icaros. Seizing the momentary strength, I called out again, even more declaratively. "Ayudame, hermanos." Help me. Help me, brothers.

I was fading hard and fast. The darkness was starting to

engulf my being. I was now the embodiment of the orb of light that I had seen earlier, and I was now facing a very real darkness that sought to oust me and take hold of my body.

As blackness took hold of my vision, I could hear the shuffling of feet and muttering from Jose, Horatio, and Kelly growing nearer. I even got a brief glimpse of a headlamp as they reached my mat and began to try and support my now weakening body. My consciousness waned, waxed slightly, and waned again. I muttered to my rescuers solely in Spanish. It was as if I had no choice to speak in English.

The war waged on, feeling as if it was a war over my body but one that had to be fought solely by my spirit. I was utterly bewildered by what my assailant was and where it had come from. It was completely unfamiliar to me, something that I had not been previously harboring and had zero experience with, and consequently left me desperate to find a way to defend against it. I wasn't sure if it was just my memory, but I could almost hear the half-voice that Zach and I had witnessed earlier. Both were equally dark and alluded to a great deal of power that I wasn't fully able to comprehend.

I collapsed to the wooden floor of the maloca and gasped for a metaphorical lungful of air during a moment where I glimpsed my physical surroundings. I was slumped over near the bathroom, utterly confused as I had wholeheartedly believed that I was already in the bathroom. A surge of animosity filled me in my desperation, my head swimming as I tried to reconcile my reality.

I was being supported by several arms, none of which

seemed to be connected to the bodies that came to my aid. The beam of a headlamp shone over me as someone brought me some water. I could vaguely hear the shaman hovering over me and chanting, and my panicked desperation only grew, as I felt their healing powers were futile and inadequate. It seemed I was truly the only one that could help myself. Beads of icy sweat were streaking down my hot cheeks as havoc was reeked on my stomach; a tempest was brewing in my belly.

"El baño. Quiero sentarme en el baño," I adamantly told those around me. I needed to sit upright, and the closest seat was the toilet several feet to my right. Noticing my newfound urgency, I was assisted to my feet and escorted to sit on the porcelain.

Despite my lack of physical control of my body, I was able to get my pants around my ankles, bracing myself to expel something in an attempt to save myself. My rescuers had all retreated beyond the bathroom doorway to attend to the others, except Kelly who placed a bucket, a headlamp, and a water bottle within arm's reach of me before saying "I'll be right outside" and latching the door behind him.

Still blacking out, my tormentor continuously attempted to gain ground as I fought to retain a connection between my body and mind. A surge of nausea in my belly caused me to reach out for the bucket and put my sweaty, gaunt face in its opening and vomit into its depths. The umbral bathroom was suffocating me and I reached out for the headlamp with my free hand, the other still clutching the bucket.

I found the power button that lit the headlamp with my

trembling index finger, producing a dim, purple hued light. I expected for the light to produce relief, but instead my warped perspective made the bathroom appear incredibly vast. Its tiled walls seemed to extend several meters away from me, giving me the sense that I was in a dark geometric prison and alienated from any help and the world that lay just beyond the door.

Another surge of darkness caused my stomach to turn. I again heaved into the bucket, emptying my stomach of its viscous contents. My body felt so distanced from myself that I was unsure if vomitus had splashed back onto my face or shirt, but the thought quickly passed as I realized that was the least of my worries now. The smell of death and shit still clung to the air and was constantly prodding at my gag reflex.

The sense of being forsaken was incredibly overwhelming and my thoughts again turned to Christ's solitary suffering in Gethsemane. I summoned enough strength to call out and ensure that someone was still outside. I wasn't sure if it was a conscious decision due to Kelly's horrible grasp of the Spanish language, but I finally called out in English.

"Kelly, are you still there?"

A moment passed before I received affirmation of his presence. "Yeah, I'm here buddy," he said. I could not spend another minute in this prison, isolated with only my dark attacker. "Would you come in here and just be a presence for a minute. He obliged and stood in the dark corner. As I continued to reel in my torment, I saw him with a look of slight discomfort of being in the bathroom with me. I couldn't blame him. The reason I had respite from what are normally uncomfortable boundaries was that I was instead focusing on fighting for my soul, my mind, my consciousness.

Now realizing that I was not in any danger of diarrhea, I struggled to pull my pants back up to my waist. Another twinge in my gut reared its head.

"How are you doing, man?" Kelly asked from the corner as I slumped over with my glistening face cradled in a shaky hand. I looked side to side, vivid tracers moving across my field of vision as I did so, almost as if I was answering with a desperate shake of my head. And that answer would have been fairly accurate.

At this point my frustration and confusion were at an all-time high, as I struggled to reconcile the origin and meaning of the war I was waging. I told Kelly I had no idea how I was and expressed my utter confusion, mentioning how I had never experienced any sort of crisis like this before and how I was scrambling to try and find a way to manage it.

For a moment, I began to worry that I may never be able to bring myself to do psychedelics again. This venture into the unknown was making me reconsider my ability to manage my reality under such vulnerable circumstances.

Kelly was surprised when he found out that I had gone up for a second and third cup, letting out a slow "Oh, yeah... You're going to be high for a looooong time, buddy." His attitude rubbed me the wrong way. It was a comforting reminder that I was high and that ultimately things would give way to "normalcy," but at the same time it was slightly insensitive trying to declare this existential war I was taking part in as strictly the product of a "high." Either way, I had no time to linger on such trivialities. He stayed for a moment longer before leaving once more to attend to the other participants.

Once more I reached for the puke bucket as my stomach surged. I was half afraid that the bucket may overflow, but in the light of my headlamp I glimpsed the frothy bile only taking up half of its volume. Half empty. "No, half full," I said to myself. In this battle, perspective and attitude was going to dictate my fate.

My blackouts were slowly starting to be less intense and less frequent, and the longer I sat in the bathroom, the more I wanted to leave. Finally deeming myself fit to return to my mat, I stood up and walked to the bathroom door. There was a dull thud and a creek as my fingers found the latch and began to swing the door open on its hinges.

I was immediately bathed in the soft, familiar, orange glow of the candle in the middle of the room. It stood with such a strong identity, with a triumphant, living light that felt impervious to the darkness. Kelly was still standing as a silhouette next to the bathroom door, his cap and ponytail distinct in the dancing candlelight.

He turned toward me and put a gentle hand on my shoulder before saying "Welcome back, Captain." I remembered that one of my early grade school gym teachers always called me Captain Stu. I thanked him. Still unsteady, I slowly stepped across the floor into the circular arrangement of mats. Somehow I truly felt as though I had left my "crew" and "ship" behind, embarking on a peril filled adventure where I was forced to make do without their love and support. Several of them were already sitting upright on their mats, coming out of their visions. They seemed to watch me as I made my way back to my seat.

The battle was not yet won, but I had gained some ground. Being enveloped in the light of the candle gave me something to ground myself with, gaining strength from being present in my body and mind, as I devotedly gazed into the flame. I tried to re-posture myself to physically reinforce this centeredness, crossing my legs, and straightening my back.

The respite from my torment was only temporary. Suddenly, the darkness surged again. Almost as if aware that it was losing its grip on me, it reared back for another full-fledged attack.

My body once again became weak and I was engulfed in despair. I looked right and left at Zach and Shayne, but both seemed to still be quite preoccupied with their meditations with Ayahuasca, but Kim was sitting soberly just beyond. Instantly, I knew I needed Kim's help. As my arms and voice began to shake, I got up the courage to speak.

"I know this is a strange request," faltered my voice, "but I feel like I really need to be close to my family now. Zach, Shayne, and Kim, if any of you are comfortable with it, it would help me a lot if you guys came and just sat next to me."

Almost immediately, Kim began to rise and walk over to my mat. I knew that Zach and Shayne weren't able or ready to come to my aid, and I forgave them, merely wishing they were going through less suffering than I was. Kim sat down to my right and slightly behind me. From across the room, Cole also rose from his mat and walked over to mine to sit on my left side.

In the midst of my grappling, I requested that they each

place a hand on my back near my heart. Both happily obliged and I could immediately feel their warmth giving me strength. Kim's hand moved in a soothing and motherly circle, while Cole's stayed firm and unmoving. I felt as though I had finally found my grounding, almost as if I had been dialed into a state of perfect receptiveness. My posture was impeccably strong and my mind was clear and pointed, as I slowly turned my head and gazed wide-eyed and alert around the room.

An overwhelming surge, one of equal intensity to the one that had initially fallen upon me, coursed through every fiber of my Being. However, this time it was a surge of complete love. It warmed me, casting a radiant glow into the darkness. This was what godliness was. The outpouring of love from, and for, these two individuals quickly made tears well in my eyes. I was witnessing and experiencing absolute divinity from these two mortals who came so selflessly to my aid.

Shaken by the tsunami of love I was experiencing, I struggled to find my voice and words that appropriately demonstrated how much I loved and appreciated Cole and Kim. My voice shook and my words felt as though they were incredibly inadequate of conveying the degree of love I felt. I hoped that they could just feel it radiating from my heart, through their hands, and straight to their own hearts. "I've never believed in guardian angels before, but this is what I imagine it feels like. You guys have saved me," I said with a quavering voice. They both told me that they loved me too.

I felt another pang of nausea, and quickly grabbed my bucket and tilted forward in an attempt to shield my saviors.

Their hands stayed firm on my back. I felt almost sucked out of my body. When I spewed into the bucket there was an eerie sense of dissociation as the vomit fell from my mouth.

Kelly walked over to me with another bottle of water, which I drank from, even if only to rinse my mouth.

As Cole sat channeling healing energy which he had been shown in the night before, he asked about what I was going through. I paused before telling him that I had been fighting a violent war over my soul, that a darkness was seeking to oust me from my body. It was then that he said something so striking and something that resonated so hard within me. He looked into my eyes with and spoke with a grave tone. "We are the lucky ones. We get to have bodies."

Coming from a Mormon upbringing, I had been taught in church that one third of all spirits had been denied the opportunity to receive corporeal bodies; these spirits were forever resentful of the other two thirds and coveted their bodies above all else, and often sought to beguile those spirits with bodies into physical vulnerability. Despite the never-ending list of my grievances over Mormon doctrines, never had such a concept felt so possible.

Now that he knew a bit more about what I was dealing with, Cole further encouraged me to draw upon our conversation from earlier that morning. He advised me to declare "I am." I hesitated a moment to summon all of my focus and energy before finally gazing into the flame of the candle. "I AM." It was not even just meant as "I am," but as to formally address my assailant that "I am, and I am not yours." This statement only added to the bastion of support that I was receiving, continuing to show glistening hope in my struggle.

As Cole felt me easing under his and Kim's hands, his relentless sense of humor began to show its head. He began making jokes about the fictional new TV drama we had created called *Safari Jack*, a show following the antics of "a loose-cannon park ranger named Jack" that foiled the plots of poachers and was full up to his fedora with safari puns. We all were at the mercy of Cole's barrage of jokes that quickly put us in stitches. The fact that I could laugh again was a good sign.

Several people were starting to chat as the curanderos bid us goodnight. It seemed as though no one was in any particular rush to leave the maloca.

I was still experiencing swells while we sat together. Someone called out in surprise, as a fairly large tarantula made its way into the light of the candle and crawled toward their mat. Surprised, we all shifted in our places in unease. The spider was ten feet from me, but it immediately began to cause me a great deal of distress. I was not afraid for my safety but certainly was not ready to have to think about such a presence as I sat trying to maintain a calm composure. As a few people gathered around it, the tarantula made a quick dart and I asked if we could do something about the spider. "Please don't kill it, but can we somehow move it away from here?" I by no means wanted to witness a death in my current state, but merely wanted relief from its presence. Kelly found an empty bucket and placed it over the spider to at least put it out of sight and limit its mobility.

Finally, Shayne moved closer to join our family huddle. Kim

and I began talking about music festivals, our drug experiences, and about Caitlin and my history. As someone that I had not met prior to our trip to Peru, I was quickly growing quite fond of Kim. She may as well have been a blood relative that I had known for most of my life. I told Shayne that he was a lucky guy to have Kim in his life, to which he promptly replied, "Oh, trust me. I know."

Surrounded by my family, my love for them grew exponentially. Each one of them was now considered one of my dearest friends, ones that I hoped to keep for the rest of our lives.

My battle was clearly coming to a close, with me as the triumphant victor. As I began to try to analyze and interpret my experiences, I was unable to shake a number of resounding similarities to stories I had heard in my religious upbringing. Considering my apostasy from any organized religion and general disdain for its agendas, I was puzzled by how my experiences spoke to those frameworks. Was I about to reshape my concept of spirits and religion? I nervously tried to put it out of mind for the time being.

After several more minutes in the maloca, Zach, Shayne, Kim, and I decided we were ready to leave and go back as a family to Zach and my bungalow. We gathered our things and embarked into the darkness.

Shayne and Zach decided to fetch a couple of extra blankets and pillows from Shayne and Kim's bungalow, one of the furthest from the maloca, leaving Kim and I to talk. I sat in the hammock, gently swaying in the light of the candle as she sat in the rigid, wooden chair.

We spoke about how great it was having a smaller group here in the jungle compared to the group of eighteen that we had been a part of earlier in our trip, laughing at the idea of how unprepared the two blonde girls from the group would be in the jungle. Our conversation then shifted to talking about our families and siblings. Kim talked about how annoying and rude it is being an adult in their thirties and having everyone always ask when they were going to start popping out children, as if that's the only purpose to exist. We took turns in voicing our agreement on how crucial it is for parents to be able to balance a finite amount of time and attention to children, and dividing that time up into smaller, disproportionate pieces as they bring more children into the world. At some point it becomes a selfish act. To have one or two kids but still feel that they are not enough? An absurdly ungrateful thought.

My two cousins returned safely and we sat quietly conversing for an hour as Zach played intricate melodies on the guitar, his fingers sounding even more articulate on the fret board than usual. Kim started to drift off to sleep as we were kept awake and alert, still processing each of our experiences. After an hour, Shayne and Kim decided to make the trek to sleep in their own bungalow. We each hugged one another and voiced our love for one another before they embarked.

Zach and I returned to our seats and enjoyed a few moments of silence before either of us spoke. Surprisingly, it was Zach who broke the silence first.

He slowly turned to me and with a low voice said "This is

between us for right now, but I have a theory on what happened tonight." I voiced my vow of disclosure before Zach continued. He began to talk about his feelings that he and I had a joint experience tonight, fighting the same demon. A list of crazy coincidences from the night's proceedings came to fall into an unnervingly cohesive theory that supported the timeline in which the presence we heard and sensed outside our bungalow, Horatio's staring outside the maloca just before ceremony began, how the generator power had cut off just as Jose had extinguished the candles and plunged the entire compound into darkness, and the number of individual healings that occurred that night.

My body filled with buzzing energy, as the depth of this theory came to be fully realized in my mind. Zach theorized that we had each taken part in exorcising a darkness that someone we loved had been harboring; a great darkness that they did not yet have the tools or experience to conquer without it destroying them. It was the combination of our mutual love for this person and our experiences that gave us the capacity to undertake this mission on their behalf. This idea only reinforced my earlier thoughts that I was experiencing a torment that I could not tackle without the help of Cole and Kim, and sent jolts of buzzing electricity through my extremities.

What an incredibly beautiful concept, that acts of love allow us to help others conquer their darkest moments that they cannot vanquish completely on their own. This act alone is our highest calling as human beings, to be redeemers of our fellow beings. Isn't that what made Jesus so remarkable? Being part human and part divine, he supposedly suffered and died for the sins of all, something that no other was able to do for humanity, and redeem us all. We may be born gods, but we are not born redeemers.

We talked about the correlations between what we were experiencing here and the religious framework that we had each grown up with. Acknowledging the bit of truth in the common Christian phrase "Faith without works is dead," it became clear that it was our preparation in readying our Selves that allowed us to be able to tackle someone else's burden. In each of our lives, there will come a time where we are called upon to do something for another who is unable to do so for themselves. It is our job to make sure that we are adequately prepared to undertake the sacrifice. Without being sound in our own Selves, it is next to impossible for us to be capable of not being shaken by the weight and struggle of the task of bearing another's grave burden.

Our eyes glowed wide with amazement in the dim candlelight as we took turns, seemingly spewing revelatory truths. After several minutes, our conversation took a pause and we each seemed to take a big breath as the gravity of our words amalgamated in our minds.

I had spoken in tongues earlier. It may not have been in a dead or dying language, but in my most desperate hour of need I had managed to speak a language other than my first with astounding authority, given the situation. Zach told me how shocked he was when he first heard me call out in the darkness and heard me continue to speak while I collapsed and regained consciousness. With his lack of any Spanish skills, I'm sure it sounded even more like a bizarre, non-terrestrial tongue.

Still reeling in the lucidity that I found occupying my mind, I began to notice congruencies between my experience and the body of art that I had begun before coming to Peru. Conceptually, this new body of work was exploring the physical and existential natures of light and darkness and how they are related to practices of ceremony and ritual. As I stared at the flickering flame of the candle, I realized that I had landed myself in the perfect opportunity to learn about these ideas first hand.

In writing about this new body of work, I had written about the world in which the first humans had lived at the mercy of light and darkness, two magnanimous entities which dominated early man's physical and spiritual existence. Darkness was, and still remains, the natural state of things. Light must be created and cultivated, where darkness merely is and always will be. Although, despite its dazzling beauty and complexity, and even its often-violent tendencies, Nature itself is inherently morally void. It is up to individuals to generate light, casting new knowledge and awareness out of the shadows of the uncertain and the unknown. In order to truly know the light, I had to experience absolute darkness, both physically and spiritually. I had already been cast into the dense, physical darkness that so thickly blankets the Amazon when the sun sets, but now I had been thrust into the spiritual abyss. I had seen the other side, and made it back.

I suddenly knew that this dance with darkness was the reason I was meant to burn my ceremonial clothes. It was as if the bleached white garments had been soiled and desecrated, now possibly harboring scattered remnants of darkness in their fibers.

Zach and I continued to talk through the night talking about the implications of the night's ceremony, taking note in the sky's transition from a deep navy to lighter shades of red, orange, purple. As the night shift were returning to their nests and burrows, the Amazon's day shift began to call out in the fresh morning air announcing their awakening. As light started to peek through the foliage, we put on our rubber boots and began walking to the dock where we had arrived.

We descended a long series of wooden steps down to the wooden dock. The soft morning light reflected off the glassy surface of the river, the green leaves becoming brighter as the sun climbed higher. We sat in two handcrafted chairs made from reclaimed materials and gazed across the water, watching fish jump to snatch tiny insects hovering just above the surface.

As I followed the gentle ripples radiating outward, I couldn't help but realize how impossible it is to feel alone in the Amazon. The reminders that life, in all its forms, is all around you and constant. It was a realization that simultaneously brought solace and disquiet, but ultimately, I was just incredibly grateful that I had Zach with me. I wouldn't have been alone without him, but his presence was an incredibly comforting one. After quietly contemplating the night's events for several moments, I joked that we were going to have to write a "bible."

Zach and I continued to watch the sunrise over the tree tops until we heard the rustling of cookware up the hill, as the cocineras began to prepare our morning bowls of fruit. The thought of fresh banana and papaya made my stomach growl, but a massive yawn reminded me that I was in dire need of sleep.

We climbed the stairs with heavy, tired feet and made our way back to our bungalow in relative silence. Before climbing into our mosquito-netted beds, I gave Zach a big hug, told him I loved him, and thanked him for being there throughout the crazy night.

My eyelids began to take on an unimaginable weight as I slowly clambered up the steep series of planks that led to the second floor of the bungalow. As I walked to my bed, I caught a glimpse of two large spider molts that had fallen from the vaulted ceiling, but was too preoccupied with exhaustion to bat an eye. With eyes closed, I reached out to find the opening in the mosquito net canopy and practically careened onto my bed. Sleep had never come so quickly.

A full day had passed since the last ceremony. We had woken up from our second night with the Medicine weary, in both body and mind, and all realized why the Refugio took a break from ceremony every third day.

On the fourth day, I woke to the gentle sound of a rain shower. I stirred under the red and gold blanket that I had buried my head under to escape the night time jungle. The pitter-patter of water droplets bombarding the broad leaves of the rainforest canopy was a far less jarring wakeup call than the car alarms in Lima, allowing me to ease back into waking life.

After several minutes enjoying the rain, I climbed out of bed and stealthily descended the stairs. Zach continued to sleep deeply, while my bare feet fell silently on each step and over to the main door and unlatched it. I took extra care to lift the door slightly as I swung it on its hinges.

I was filled with disappointment to find that small, black ants had found their way under the plastic wrap on our fruit bowls and had beat us to the feast. Begrudgingly, I removed the plastic coverings and tossed the colorful cubes of fruit on the forest floor. "Let the ants have it," I told myself, "they need it more than you."

For the past twenty-four hours, I had been fiercely debating whether or not I would participate in tonight's ceremony. My second meditation with Ayahuasca had been far more intense than I could have ever imagined, and had shaken me enough to consider not partaking in the Medicine again. But today was a new day and my hesitation of the previous day was starting to give way. My work was not done and there was so much more for me to learn. Besides, how could this next ceremony be even more intense than what I had already survived?

My mind was made up. I needed to partake. Only this time I would be patient, trusting in Jose's judgment and in the dose of Medicine that he deemed right for me.

Again, we spent our day filling time between our meals of chicken, rice, and lentils with naps, reading, and games. Engrossing my mind in an intense game of Liar's Dice with Cole, Curtis, and my cousins kept it from dwelling on my anxiety about the upcoming ceremony. I kept telling myself that there was no way that tonight would be worse than the second night, but then again, how could I know that for sure?

The afternoon came and went and once again I found myself gathering my wits about me in preparation for another night of learning and upheaval. This time I was not going to don my white clothes, which I had been keeping in exile outside the bungalow like a leper. Whether you call it a newfound superstition or just taking every possible precaution, I dug through my bag for a shirt and the Incan scarf that the shaman Augostin had blessed at the water temple in Urqos. I rummaged in the dim lamp light, passing up my shirt from a band called Full of Hell, and pulled out a dark red, Touché Amoré shirt. The idea that having a form of the word 'love' printed on the shirt gave me a bit of peace of mind.

Downstairs, I sat and fiddled with the Incan cross that hung from my neck, touching each of the twelve points contemplatively as Zach gathered his effects for ceremony. As I sat, I knew that tonight I needed to ask Ayahuasca to be gentle with me in helping me fulfill my intention; I wanted tonight to be manageable, and that would require that I be more specific and targeted.

Once again, a Guardian came to retrieve us and lead us to the maloca. I sat and focused on controlling my breath, being present in every inhale and exhale in an attempt to calm my nerves. Familiar faces appeared in the doorway and took their spots at their usual mats. I smiled at humans' apparent tendency to claim a space for their own and consistently return to it without instruction to do so.

The two curanderos showed up together. Jose's white embroidered vest gave off a soft glow in the darkness. After briefly speaking to someone else in the group, Jose made his way over to where I sat.

"Como estas, mi hermano?" he said lightly with a gentle smile that seemed to already know the answer. I was flattered that such a spiritual man had so fondly called me his brother.

"Muy bien. Mucho mejor," I told him, reflecting his calming tone.

Despite my feelings that the curanderos were truly unable to comprehend my previous torment and sufficiently come to my aid, Jose reassured me that he knew exactly what had been going on. Of course he did, I told myself. How could such a mystic not know after working intimately with the Medicine for upwards of thirty years.

He knew that I was entering uncertain territory where I would be vulnerable when I came up to him asking for a second and third sacrament, but I was already with the Medicine, and he was not to interfere. His wisdom was great, but Ayahuasca's is still more vast and intuitive. We gave each other a firm, brotherly embrace and he smiled as he patted me on the shoulder before going to prepare the ceremony materials.

As the preparations were made, Shayne finally brought to my attention just how brief the ceremonies lasted. I was shocked to find that the curanderos had been leaving the maloca each night around 11 p.m. and on the night of our second ceremony we had returned to our bungalow at 11:45 p.m. How could all of my torment have been condensed into a mere three hours? The Medicine clearly did not abide by the same time table as the rest of reality. Hours may just as well have been days.

Conversation died out among our group. The ritual was the same, as always. Sanctify. Partake. Protect. Bless. The Ayahuasca seemed to taste even more acrid than before and almost made me sputter after I drank from the small cup. I silently hoped the increasing bitterness of the Medicine was not some kind of omen.

Jose came around to each of us with the Agua de Florida, marking our foreheads, hands, and hearts. Unlike the taste of the Ayahuasca, I was becoming more and more fond of the floral odor of the Agua and looked forward to each time Jose came around to me to bless me by gently blowing tiny droplets of it onto the top of my head.

I sat breathing deeply, admiring the consistency and rigorous precautions taken with each ceremony with a newfound respect in securing the space and ensuring a safe experience for all participating. Kelly had told us over lunch the previous day about large outdoor parties where people had been drinking Ayahuasca and having massive orgies. The idea of such reckless behavior without the proper supervision of a shaman was mind boggling. I could only imagine what kind of darkness could take advantage of a situation like that where so many were left so vulnerable.

The familiar fluttering of leathery bat wings zipped past my ear as I began to focus on conscious breathing and solidifying the night's intention.

After having such an incredibly radical experience regarding my spiritual being, I decided to finally request the Medicine's insight on my practice as an artist. It was clear that my previous intention had been left too open to interpretation, and I took extra caution in selecting my words to ensure me a happier and gentler experience this time around. My lungs filled with the warm night air and the aromatic smoke of nearby mapacho, calming my anxious heartbeat as the words, "Show me the path I must take to become the best, happiest, and most fulfilled artist I can be" began to take shape in my mind.

I silently repeated the mantra, each time becoming more grateful that I had included the contingency of my lasting happiness.

With my eyes already closed, I was not aware that Jose had taken up the leaf fan and put out the candle. I was already starting to see the static darkness behind my eyelids shift and writhe like black flies. It was only a matter of time now. As I lay on my mat, I occasionally opened my eyes in nervous anticipation to glimpse the deep blue sky as a momentary reprise from the images that would soon demand my attention.

The Icaros were of a different breed tonight. The words were the same, but there was a clear difference in the sultry tone with which Jose sang them. There was a feebleness to his vibrato that made him seem like a much older version of himself.

Jose's voice continued with the inspired melodies as we all began to delve deeper into the Medicine. Slowly and subtly, it crept up almost imperceptibly. The inklings of writhing shapes continued to intensify, taking on more definite shapes. My heartbeat was now beating more distinctly; I could feel it in every fiber of my Being. It was not racing with a feverish pace, but seemed to be pumping blood very deliberately through my veins in certain anticipation.

Jose had stopped singing, giving Horatio the floor to begin the healing sessions with three individuals. Where Jose sang with a sweeping legato, Horatio's song took a more rhythmically percussive form that reminded me of the times I had heard Native American shaman sing in pow-wows and other ceremonies. It was astonishingly beautiful and I couldn't help but direct my attention to him as he sat beside those he was healing.

In a great swell, I was thrust into a vision. Initially, it was unclear if my eyes had remained open or had instinctively shut tight. I was now in a surreal space of darkness, full of fluorescent lines that began to form a geometric structure. Lines of brilliant yellow, orange, and pink converged to create a neon temple amidst the darkness. The lines seemed simple at first, creating a shallow sense of depth, but quickly began to allude to a vastness that dwarfed both me and the temple. I could not see myself within this space and seemed to float up the steps of the temple in first person, passing two large spires that stood on either side of the grand entrance.

The suddenness with which I was being immersed in this new space startled me. I immediately became reluctant to fully give in to the Medicine as I remembered how close I had felt to losing my Self when it took hold of me. I panicked slightly. I hated to admit it, but against my better judgment, I was fighting against the Medicine.

I opened my eyes to the dark maloca just as I had entered the brilliant temple. My fear of letting go had begun to manifest in my beating heart, its pace quickening with my anxious breath. I stared at the dark vaulted ceiling with my hands over my heart as I tried to comfort myself. The sound of Cole's violent vomiting traveled through the darkness and could be heard over Horatio's singing.

Feigning composure, I turned to face where Horatio was kneeling next to Kim and tried to ground myself in my physical reality. As I lay on my side it was clear that the Medicine was not going to give in so easily. The Ayahuasca surged through my extremities with a force that I had never experienced before. It had jettisoned me to a level of high that demanded that I bend to its will. Almost as if my body was a marionette, I felt compelled against my better judgment to lay on my side with my hands folded under my head and succumb.

I felt myself delve deeper into the Medicine and once again found myself in the temple, rising a second set of stairs to what I immediately knew was an altar. I began to contemplate kneeling in adoration, but once again tried to open my eyes. My eyes had hardly opened before slamming shut again, the temple disappearing.

I was now face to face with a seemingly infinite line of similarly fluorescent harpies. Each of their hybrid bodies were identical to the one on either side of it. They were reminiscent of Egyptian hieroglyphs as they moved their radiant pink wings in tandem. Each gazed at me uninterruptedly with intense faces that were equal parts human and vulture. It was a mesmerizing display of both feathers and flesh. I watched in awe, pondering if these hybrids were deities, demons, or merely sanctioned guardians of the temple I had seen.

Without any warning at all, my vision was once again interrupted as my jaw was flung open in a gaping yawn that made my entire body quake. The yawn seemed to go on and on, wider and wider as it were going to turn my head inside out. Nausea grabbed at my stomach and I became disoriented the wider my mouth opened.

Even in light of my second ceremony, I had never experienced a high like this. It was blisteringly intense, and once again made me question if I could manage its power. Breathe. Just breathe.

After what seemed like an eternity, my mouth finally fell closed. Even as my lips pressed together in relief, silent, creeping tears began to pour from my eyes. Despite the disorienting intensity of the Medicine, I knew that these were not tears of sadness. My chest did not heave with sobs and my breath did not falter. I had to reach a hand to my face and trace the wet lines with my quivering fingertips to believe that they were streaming so consistently down my cheeks. As I wiped my tears on my shirt, I grabbed my bucket and placed it next to me as if to brace for a more violent purging to come.

Another cataclysmic yawn took hold of me, ushering a new stream of tears as I witnessed a panther come to me out of the darkness. Its lean body was blacker than night itself, reflecting a deep, dark purple in the moonlight of my mind as it strode to perch itself on a rock. Its body lurched and from its fierce jaws sprang a fountain of bright white that cascaded into a pool of water below. The panther's yellow eyes squeezed shut and the pool became illuminated by its glowing vomitus. It struck me as odd that this messenger was the one emptying its stomach and not me.

The panther began to pan out of view as I followed the flow of the glowing liquid to an opposite shore. A majestic and heavily ornamented bull stood on the dark bank, and slowly proceeded to wade into the shallows and meet the luminous current. The red and gold headdress that rested on his great white head did not fall as he bowed to the water's surface and began to lap up the beaming water with a heavy, violet tongue.

The bull's dark eyes closed heavily, his velvet muzzle hovering over the surface of the water. He was clearly as unthreatened by the nearby panther as I was. His great throat undulated as peristalsis forced the liquid down his esophagus. As the bull drank, he seemed to radiate an increasingly bright aura of divinity into the surrounding darkness.

Another cavernous yawn forced a new wave of salty tears to stream down my face, and in its wake my eyes crept open for a brief moment, giving me a glimpse of the darkened maloca. The tranquility of my vision was not reflected in my perceived control of my corporeal experience, as I thought to myself "I have never been high like this before."

In the moments where I tried to stave off the bold advances that the Medicine was making on my being, I tried to find the ability to remove myself from the visions. Each time the Ayahuasca fought back, pulling me back to lay on my mat with an intense, supernatural strength. The reminders that I was in the hands of a force much wiser and stronger than myself were constant, and ultimately forced me to bend to its will for my own benefit.

Once I decided to fully succumb, my mind erupted. In an instant, my mind became inundated with validations and knowledge about itself and its unbridled potential. The knowledge being bestowed upon me was crystal clear and pure. I came to truly understand my brain, and the brains of all others, as not only an organ, but as a conduit which allows us to experience reality.

As individuals go through the journey of life, it is our minds that assimilate all sensory information about ourselves and the world that we encounter, taking in all we see, smell, taste, hear, feel, and learn. From this raw information, our mind constructs our own uniquely subjective representations, metaphorical facsimiles of the objective reality of our existences. Metaphor is the language of the mind after all, facilitating the comprehension of ideas that are so much vaster than our own finite realms of experience

A boy riding on the back of a great polar bear, pointing towards the starry heavens and visages of young adolescents having intimate, unspoken meditations with different animals began to appear, warp, and disappear, as knowledge continued to funnel into my liberated mind.

From what we glean from objective reality, each of our own existences is entirely in our control to shape as we please. Bias, the fallibility of memory, and our unbridled creativity driven by imagination distort, revise, and embellish the subjective worlds that we choose to live in. Our mediation of our subjective reality and the objective reality is what truly defines us.

The words "it's all in your head" became unavoidable in my mind, as I saw a young girl sitting across from a monkey, both tenderly clasping hands in the light of a lantern in a silent exchange of understanding. I heard this phrase so often used in a negative manner to dismiss one's thoughts and feelings, diminishing the true capabilities of our minds. Yes, it is all in our heads. Everything: our realities, our memories, thoughts, and experiences, our figments of imagination, and the incredible capacity to change the circumstances of our lives.

As we find ourselves in an unending flood of information, our mind creates stories, associations, and metaphors that allow us to construct these worlds of existence. The true power of this process lies in how we utilize these to either empower or disenfranchise our Selves in the journey of life. Existence is not just about what you have received, but what you choose to do with what you have been given.

Choice. The creation of life and existence is the product of conscious choice; the mind, in all its beautiful and infinite complexity even allows us to dream up completely fictional worlds far removed from our realms of experience. We can build worlds and even get to decide which we choose to exist in at any given moment. But with this power comes the responsibility to be mindful that our choices to do so have repercussions that will greatly affect us.

Amidst the buzzing of my brain, to my right I could hear Shayne purge quietly into his bucket. I silently expressed my gratitude for my purging taking on the form of body shaking yawns and silent tears.

As if struck by a bolt of white-hot clairvoyance, I was made aware of my true nature and calling as an artist: the power, and even innate responsibility, to create fictional realms to inform others of 'truths' about our own world like so many artists, authors, storytellers, and other creative minds have done before. So clear was the realization of the artist as a sort of mystic or shaman whose duty it is to bridge the gap between higher realms of illumination, enlightenment, and mankind. But how does the artist make this tangible and accessible to others?

My question seemed incredibly dumb and was immediately answered. I was already doing it, and doing it as I lay in the maloca surrounded by the vast Amazon jungle. Living. Not just existing, but truly living with purpose and seeking new knowledge and greater perspective through experiences was the answer.

Scenes of adventures in faraway places began to swarm my field of vision. Riding bikes through the hills of Italy on beautiful summer nights, filling the warm night air with laughter as we passed rustic, tile-roofed villas. I could actually feel the cool rush of the breeze on my face. Lovers then walked hand in hand on a golden beach, waves lapping at the sand as a crimson sun began to dip below the horizon. It is moments like these, ecstatic realizations of true happiness and adventure that we as living beings so inherently and desperately seek. The desire to truly live runs through each one of us.

My trip to Peru had been a long string of these glorious moments. This pilgrimage was a literal odyssey of enlightenment and fulfillment, a crucial opportunity for me to truly glow as an individual. The opportunity had presented itself to me, and to my great fortune I had prepared myself to take full advantage of it, but one doesn't merely stumble upon a happy and fulfilled life full of opportunities for growth.

A break in Horatio's healing Icaros and the quick beam from Jose's flashlight jarred my eyes open and broke my trance, but only for a quick second.

Like all forms of creation, the cultivation of a happy life full of fertile opportunities for growth requires dedicated work and conscious decisions. Good things are never free. They demand investment and sacrifice, and truly great things often require even more. Happiness is ultimately a choice that we each have to make, one that we must make on a daily basis.

Prior to leaving for Peru, I had been frugal with my money, ensured that I bought the proper equipment, and made arrangements to keep my job secure – physical and material preparations. Once I arrived in South America, we were immersed in environments that provided us with spiritual preparation. Cole and Andy had organized a yoga retreat in the Sacred Valley that focused on the practices of grounding and conscious intention, both of which would prove to remain recurring themes throughout our trip. We had gone to visit and experience the spiritual haven of Machu Picchu and were inspired by both the Incan people's unity with the Earth and cosmos and their technological prowess, as they constructed such an awe-inspiring marvel. We even had the benefit of encountering several other shamans whose connection to all things and intuitive wisdom continued to leave us speechless time and time again.

Even as all these preparations seemed like adventures unto themselves, they were all vital to the preparation for what we would experience in the Amazon. I was thoroughly convinced that my experience with Ayahuasca would have been radically different if I had not prepared as I did.

Just as my heart began to beat with a quickening pace, I heard the soft sound of Jose's bare feet crossing the wooden floor, then the sound of a flint being struck as a miniscule flame appeared in the center of the room and jumped to consume the wick of the white candle.

I sat up, quickly and almost entirely without thinking. It was as if the light of the candle was compelling me to come back and center myself back into both my physical body and the maloca. My head spun a bit as I sat upright, crossing my legs in hopes to steady myself. I had tracers again. I peered about the dim room, which looked as though each object had an ethereal other slightly offset from it. I saw two candles where I knew there was just one.

Many of the others had responded to the enticing call of the candlelight. Cole, Andy, Curtis, and my cousins all looked dazed as they adjusted to the light and divine, their white clothes each giving off an angelic glow. I felt my eyes widen with a gaze that sought to peer beyond the corporeal reality that lay before me.

My body felt heavy and my mind remained in an elated state of liberation. Some invisible force drew my legs to kneel and bring my chest to fall slowly down until my forehead touched the synthetic blue plastic of the mat.

After a moment, I slowly rose back upright. As we all sat immersed in the candlelight, I thought to myself that I may never encounter a place so sacred and so spiritually inspired for the rest of my days. It didn't seem real. Or at least like it could exist in our terrestrial world. The walls of the maloca seemed to disappear, as the orange glow of the candle failed to illuminate the boundaries of their wooden planks. We were like great sages basking in a powerful and eternal light.

The earthy aroma of a lit mapacho filled the air and tickled my nostrils with tiny tendrils. It was Shayne's. I turned to him and asked how he was. He gave a couple slow, pensive nods as he held the mapacho to his mouth and then uttered "I'm good." He said it in an ambiguous tone that really didn't provide any more information, but given the intense nature of Ayahuasca, I figured that response was about as good as any.

I then turned to my left and checked on Zach. He was still laying on his back, his hands folded behind his head, not saying anything, but his bewildered eyes said it all. Fifteen seconds later, he said "I'm alright" in a voice that was barely audible, even in the near silence of the maloca. Clearly he had gone through a wringer this time as well.

Jose and Horatio said their gentle goodbyes as they left to go find their own bungalows for the night. Still enraptured by the candle, I hadn't noticed that Danielle had brought out her guitar and began playing a tune as she sang, bringing yet another layer of beauty to the night. I didn't recognize the song, and given her prowess with both instruments, I figured that it was a song that she herself had written. It was beautiful and so appropriate for the environment that we were in.

After another fifteen minutes, we each began rising to our feet and preparing to venture back into the jungle. With difficulty, I found my rubber boots and nearly fell over several times attempting to slide my feet down into them. I laughed at my debilitated equilibrium and pictured myself as a newborn giraffe trying to stand on its shaky, stilt-like legs.

Warm embraces were in order, as we embarked each with our respective Guardians down the stairs and into the darkness.

I continued to struggle with my balance as Zach and I crossed the muddy terrain and vocalized my appreciation for not having a longer hike back.

We settled with our blankets in our prospective spots in the wooden arm chair and hammock. Zach procured his iPhone in an attempt to fill the bungalow with familiar music to drown out the lively and unsettling symphony of the jungle.

Zach lit the white candle on the table with his lighter before using it to spark a Canadian cigarette. I was given the honor of selecting the first several songs, but was frustratingly dazzled by the glowing touch screen that displayed an extensive music library that I struggled to navigate. Eventually, my wide eyes found the song Machu Picchu by the Strokes and thought it was rather fitting.

As the first percussive guitar harmonies rang through the small speaker, it was apparent just how warped my sense of time was. The fairly fast tempo of the song seemed to have been amped up by about fifty percent. My confusion must have been clear on my dumbfounded face, as Zach quickly took note and asked if I was alright.

We continued to peer into the flame of the candle as the Clash and Phantogram were added to the chorus of the nocturnal jungle. Never had a single, solitary flame appeared so alive; I gave myself up to its mesmerizing radiance. I slouched in the wooden chair, my troubled mind attempting to reconcile my experiences from my last two ceremonies.

The torment that I experienced as I waged for my soul on the second night felt so incredibly real and fully instigated by an external force, but in tonight's experience, Aya assured me that the mind is a metaphorical realm which casts an uncomfortable doubt into my mind. Had I really experienced the sort of entity that I had heard so much about and suffered at its hand? Or was it a metaphorical phenomenon facilitated by the incredible intuition of Mother Ayahuasca for my personalized learning? And if it was a device of Aya's teaching, did that make my experience less legitimate?

My gaze found its way over to Zach who was lounging pensively in the hammock across the room. He seemed to be searching the great beyond for answers to a question plaguing his mind. After a gentle prod, he told me that his whole night had been a harrowing experience of a reality completely filled with snakes. I silently expressed my gratitude that I had a far less terrifying conversation with the Medicine.

A sudden gust of wind burst through the trees and the bug netting that covered our bungalow, causing the flame of the candle to dance so violently that it was almost extinguished. My hopes for a night time drizzle were soon dashed as several seconds later, another gust of wind came from the opposite direction to threaten the flame once more.

How the hell does that happen? The breeze made a 180-degree turn in a matter of seconds. I may have just been super high, but it felt as though some supernatural force had a desire to snuff out the only light in the room. Our matches had gotten too damp to light during the first couple days and we had only one small lighter that was floating about in the darkness. It was only then that I realized that our candle was dwindling and we had not gotten a spare from the main compound earlier that day. Already a bit freaked out, I panicked a bit more.

Zach was already starting to doze off in the hammock and moved to sprawl out on his bed. I couldn't blame Zach for being tired. I was quite exhausted myself, but sleep was still far from reach for my buzzing brain. I definitely felt vulnerable. Every so often I would call out to him and rouse him from his rest to regain a false sense of comfort. It was the candle, the iPhone, and me versus the night – and the iPhone's battery finally hit twenty percent.

With dwindling resources, I recalled the story of the Hanukkah menorah lasting an amazing eight nights and gave a sarcastic chuckle as I thought, "What I need is a Hanukkah miracle." Even if just for my sanity's sake, I needed this single candle to last either until I drifted off or until dawn.

Aside from the sense of protection that candlelight had consistently provided for me in the jungle, I came to realize just how beautiful a soft, solitary flame is. Basking in candlelight is an incredibly intimate experience, regardless of whether you are in the dark jungle or having a romantic meal in a high-end restaurant. The mere size of the candle's flame limits the reach of its scope of illumination: you must draw near to it to experience its light and warmth. This small proximity creates a similar sense of emotional closeness to whomever you may be sharing the light with. I felt this unique intimacy each night as Zach and I returned from ceremony to gaze into the small flame as Aya continued to illuminate our minds.

Another facet of the candle's beauty that seized my attention was the impact that it had on the surrounding environment. The wooden planks that made up the table, chairs, and support beams of the bungalow looked divinely sublime in the soft orange glow and the sharp shadows that were cast across the room added a dramatic and haunting vibe within the space.

If only I could capture the beauty of these moments in an oil painting.

I called out to Zach. Several seconds passed before I repeated myself and was given a drowsy, unintelligible grunt. I knew it was lights out for him and I was now entirely on my own.

The iPhone continued to remind me of the draining battery. I began to scour the music library with songs that mentioned the jungle in the titles. I bobbed my head to the funky bass and shrill trumpet flourishes of *Jungle Fever* by Kool and the Gang. Several songs later, I found Creedence Clearwater Revival's *Run through the Jungle* and couldn't help but consider how ill-advised that would be as guidance in that moment and laugh.

Between the music and the sense of danger that the nighttime jungle instilled in me, I briefly imagined what it must have been like to suffer through the Vietnam War as member of the U.S. military. My current fears seemed well justified, but were nowhere near having the risk of being ambushed by guerrilla soldiers while I slept.

I scanned the eastern side of the tree line for hints of dawn, but only found the deep, deep blue and glimmering stars indicative of the wee hours of the morning.

A sudden yawn pried open my mouth, tilting my head back to rest on the wooden back of the chair. This was a welcomed sign. The candle was in its last moments of life and I would soon have to surrender to the darkness.

I rose from my chair, wrapped myself in my blanket, and wearily shuffled across the floor to get my headlamp. The darkness of the jungle merging with the new umbral space of the bungalow was an uncomfortable thought, and I decided to make a new, smaller space to seek refuge in.

Carefully, I lowered myself into the hammock that was now on the very edge of the candle's dying light. As I reclined in the cloth pouch, I draped my blanket over my entire body to form a cocoon-like sanctuary. Here I was free of witnessing any mysterious lights in the surrounding rainforest and less distracted by the eerie cacophony of thousands of organisms living their lives. It did in fact feel safer here, even if I was deluding myself a bit. Sleep was slow to arrive at my doorstep, but when it did, it plunged me into a sleep where even dreams could not find me.

# HONORING MY INNER GODDESS

## Psilocybin

Albert Einstein once said, "No problem can be solved from the same level of consciousness that created it." My journey of healing and reclaiming my inner goddess could not have taken place if it was not for this message. I needed to first see my own patterns and problems from an objective point of view before truly realizing how much they did not serve me.

Initially, I was inspired by MAPS' research on the use of psychedelic substances to heal mental illness. I wanted to be a part of the movement to find a means of healing for souls that truly needed it – souls much like my own, who were diagnosed with PTSD and had lost touch with their own bodies. I wanted this healing. I wanted the feeling of connectedness with my body and to love every inch of it. I just didn't know how to achieve it myself.

Opportunity knocked in the form of an eighth of mushrooms, or Psilocybe cubensis, a powerful entheogen. For those who are unfamiliar, the word entheogen means "generating God, the Divine, from within." My inner goddess was waiting for me. It was time to stop looking out and start looking in.

I consumed all of the mushrooms at once, chewing as fast as I could and hoping that something was waiting for me on the other side. I decided to play with pastels while I waited for the mushrooms to kick in. My first clue that they were becoming active in my body was the immense pleasure that I felt from the texture of the pastels, and the happiness that each individual color brought me. Following the appreciation for multiple shades of blue, my vision suddenly became high definition. I had to lie down because of the immense energy rushing through me. Every breath felt like it needed my full attention. Waves of deep pain, realization, then ecstasy rolled over me. I laid in my bed, sobbing. I cried until I couldn't feel my face anymore – rubbing my arms and legs, begging for forgiveness for not being with my body sooner.

I have been overweight for the majority of my life and thought I had been experiencing rejection from the world because of the way my body looked. It wasn't until my consciousness was altered by the mushrooms, and I felt what full presence feels like, that I realized I had been the cause of my own isolation. I had locked myself in a prison and projected judgment of myself onto others for as long as I could remember. I tried being someone else. I tried being someone else before I even knew who I was. I had been defined by the diagnoses and labels put on me, but in that moment, I was peeling back every layer of self-hatred, criticism, and trauma despite having no idea what I'd find underneath. With each layer lifted, I felt more and more forgiveness and freedom. I felt at home in my body for the first time. I don't think I had ever felt self-love before that night.

After reaching this understanding with myself after hours of discomfort, the waves of love and tranquility became much more stable. Tears of pain became tears of joy. I was home. My body was my home. This body, no matter how jiggly it is, is mine to inhabit and to cherish. My inner goddess and I had become one. The constant voice of self-doubt no longer sat in the executive seat of my mental faculty. Instead, my inner goddess, my truth, had control over my thoughts and actions. This truth shows up in my life as a greater capacity to hold space for suffering and pain, giving nothing but compassion to myself and the world around me. I couldn't believe the transition that happened within a few short hours. I simply did not feel like the same person anymore. Years of therapy could not equate to the healing and realizations I had in one eight-hour period.

I had spent my whole life living in my head and trying to ignore the fleshy meat sack that was below my chin. The mushrooms kindly redirected me to my body and connected me to my inner goddess. Instead of being an escape, I experienced a true awakening as I came face to face with my whole self; mind and body. I am in charge. This is my body. This tattoo-covered, love-filled body is mine. This is my life.

Benoit Mandelbrot, the father of fractal geometry, once said, "My life seemed to be a series of events and accidents. Yet when I look back I see a pattern." I keep those words close to my heart as I reflect on this transformational journey. Now, I can see the beautiful, complex, and colorful patterns that are my life and how my body and my inner goddess are one.

*https://www.psymposia.com/magazine/honoring-my-inner-goddess-how-mushrooms-helped-me-love-my-body/*

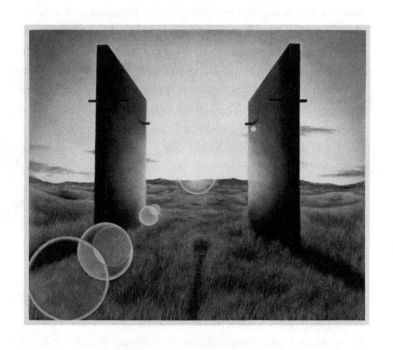

# RELAXING WITH WHAT IS

## San Pedro

I awoke to the sound of a flock of parrots flying overhead. I gave myself a nice morning stretch and stepped outside of my tent. I was located near the edge of a cliff, overlooking the beautiful Mapacho River and the Mapacho River Valley. I drank some water and headed down to the stream for a cold rinse in one of the pools.

I bathed in the gel-like substance of the San Pedro, also known as Huachuma, to clean my skin and prepare for the upcoming ceremony. The community gathered in the temple at about 8 a.m., and Roman, our shaman, spoke briefly about the Huachuma medicine and how to utilize it for healing. One of the lessons we had been learning and practicing was to simply "relax with what is." Whatever sensations we were feeling, pleasant or unpleasant, we were practicing the art of deeply relaxing into the present moment, relaxing with intensity, relaxing with discomfort, and finding peace in life's changing circumstances.

We had been following a San Pedro dieta, where you take a small amount of San Pedro each day, for a week, and today was the day that we finished our dieta with a ceremony. Before, we had been consuming the powdered form of San Pedro, but today we were going to drink a large amount of the freshly prepared medicine that we had made the previous night.

Roman invited the spirits to be with us in this ceremony,

and his wife Cynthia began beating her drum and singing a lovely song with her soothing voice. We were all sitting in a giant circle, each with our own instrument. The instruments were various types of drums and percussion instruments, as well as a few different types of shakers.

Anthony, one of Roman's apprentices, distributed the cups of San Pedro to the group, and we began drinking the thick, gelatinous and bitter liquid as we sat in our musical circle. Since we were fasting and this was our first meal of the day, Roman humorously called it, "the breakfast of champions."

We were asked not to talk to each other, but to remain quiet and to focus on our individual journeys, while also utilizing the support of the group energy. We played music and sang for about forty-five minutes as the medicine digested, and we then began the first gateway.

In the San Pedro ceremonies, there is what Roman calls "The Four Gateways," which are essentially four different practices that we do during ceremony. The first of these practices is Qigong – an ancient Chinese art which involves repetitive, slow and subtle movements to activate, tune into, and better understand the essential energy or Chi of the Universe.

We did many different Qigong practices, and the San Pedro really helped to deepen the practice. I could feel the vibrations surrounding my entire body. I was aware of the subtlest movements within me, and after some time, I could actually feel the energy coming from my hands. When I put my two hands together I felt a ball of energy, it was as if my hands had some form of repulsion, like the opposite ends of two magnets being pushed together.

There was one practice that we did that really stood out to me. We were holding our arms out at our sides with our palms facing upward, imagining that we were holding a big pot, with our head poking through a hole in the bottom of the pot – a visualization used to get the right posture. We were holding this posture for over twenty minutes. After about five minutes, my mind was starting to get restless, thinking of how difficult it was to continue holding the pose, thinking about the soreness I was feeling, thinking of excuses and reasons to quit.

As we held this pose, Roman reminded us to relax with what is, to relax with the unpleasant sensation. He said that it is these kinds of exercises which activate our secondary muscles, and the Chi that is stored in our bodies. My restless mind continued the mental chatter, desiring to give up and stop holding the pose, but I just observed it. I could strongly feel the separation between my thoughts and awareness. Dwelling in awareness I felt very peaceful, as I simply watched the behavioral patterns of my mind.

Though it didn't feel like it, apparently we had practiced Qigong for three hours! Then Roman began playing a cheerful melody on his flute, signifying that we were beginning the second gateway. The second gateway was hiking. The community I was staying with owns 4,000 acres of land, in a very remote location on the border of the Andes Mountains and the Amazon Rainforest in Peru. It was beautiful, wild, and full of life.

The group hiked barefoot down to the river, and I could really feel my connection to Pachamama (Mother Earth). As we hiked, I felt so much relaxation. I was very in-tune with the nature around me, and was in awe at the geometric patterns expressed in the different forms of plant and animal life.

I had been practicing to "relax with what is" for some time now, and the realization finally hit me. I really can be relaxed under any circumstances. I do not have to let circumstances determine my state of being, but rather I can rest in a state of total peace and relaxation, no matter what is happening. Even up until the point of death I can be relaxed, and I want to be relaxed when I die.

Realizing this, I was overcome with relaxation, happiness, and peace. I decided to sit down by the river and meditate. As I sat there, swarms of gnats, small flies, mosquitos, ants, and other insects were happy to greet me. I observed them as they landed on my exposed skin, ate their meal of human blood, and went on their way.

I didn't feel the desire to protect or defend my body, but rather I felt that everything was just Pachamama, that I myself am a part of Mother Earth, as are the insects, and I was just nourishing these sentient beings – giving back to the whole of nature, giving back to myself. I meditated for some time, and while this was a very peaceful experience, I later regretted sitting there for so long as I had plenty of fresh and itchy bug bites.

Cynthia sang some songs with her beautiful voice, one of which made me feel so free. The song was called "Pachamama," and the lyrics go:

*Pacha Mama, I'm coming home*
*To the place where I belong*
*Pacha Mama, I'm coming home,*
*To the place where I belong!*

*I want to be free, so free*
*Like the dolphin in the sea*
*Like the flowers and the bees*
*Like the birds in the trees*
*I want to fly high, so high*
*Like an eagle in the sky*
*and when my time has come*
*I'm gonna lay down and die*
*and when my time has come*
*I'm gonna rise up and fly*

*Pacha Mama I'm coming home*
*To the place where I belong*
*Pacha Mama, I'm coming home,*
*To the place where I belong!*

*I want to be free, be me*
*Be the being that I see*
*Not to rise and not to fall*

*Being one and loving all*
*There's no high*
*There's no low*

*There is no place I should go*
*Just inside a little star*
*Telling me, be as you are.*
*Just inside a little star telling me – be as you are.*

*Pacha Mama I'm coming home*
*To the place where I belong*
*Pacha Mama, I'm coming home,*
*To the place where I belong!*

After that powerful and liberating song, Roman played his flute again, and we moved onto the next gateway. This gateway was an Amazonian breathwork practice in which we do different breathing patterns for several minutes at a time. We start with our lower energy center, moving up to the energy center at our crown, and back down again.

I did this practice with my eyes closed, and with each changing breathing pattern, I also noticed different geometric patterns in my vision. Each energy center appeared to have a different mandala-like pattern associated with it. This was fascinating to see first-hand, and gave me some insight into how the ancients discovered the Chakra system and built a sacred science around it.

After the breathwork, Roman played the flute once more, and we headed up to the temple to enter into the fourth gateway. This one was very special. We were soul-gazing. Each person found a partner, and simply sat across from them and stared into each other's eyes for several minutes.

Since I had found so much peace and relaxation, I was totally at ease while staring into the eyes of my peers. I saw myself in every person. I felt so much love, so much connection, and so much beauty. I saw the very essence of life in each being, an essence that is also my own – how magical!

Others however, did not always reflect the same emotions. Some had many internal barriers, many feelings of self-judgment and lack of acceptance. I could see how challenging it was for them to be vulnerable with another human being. I saw their pain, and I saw my pain in them. I smiled, I laughed, I cried, I loved. It was so beautiful. Each person was so unique, yet the core essence was so prevalent in all of them. After each soul-gazing session there was a much needed and oh so healing hug.

We are all human beings experiencing the suffering that comes with being human: the suffering of living in our diseased society, the suffering of survival, and of coping with impermanence, emotion, and change. We are all going through this together. Why can we not always recognize this and have love for those who suffer just like we do?

So many of us choose to build barriers around our hearts to prevent ourselves from being hurt or traumatized like we were in the past. We act like we are always okay, we prevent ourselves from showing emotion, or from even feeling our emotions and some even take it to the extent of projecting their pain onto others, causing others to suffer unnecessarily. Can we not recognize these patterns of suffering? Can we not recognize the suffering within ourselves, and how we have contributed to the suffering of others?

As soon as I realized the suffering in my own life and how I was contributing to my suffering, as well as to the suffering of other beings who are really just me in another form, I cried. I felt so much guilt, shame, sorrow, and remorse. Because of my ignorance, I had hurt others. It was a terrible thing to realize. But it happened, and I accepted it. Once I accepted it, I forgave myself, and promised myself that I would do my very best to help myself and others heal, rather than perpetuate the global suffering that we have all fallen victim to, and that we all contribute to through our ignorance.

The soul-gazing really helped me to remember when I had first realized my oneness with others. Staring into the eyes of so many people so deeply, for so long, was so very healing. It helped me gain amazing insights and realizations, and also made me feel an overwhelming sense of love and belonging.

We had been fasting on nothing but San Pedro and water the whole day, and it was now very dark outside. We had made it through the four gateways together, and it was time to finish the ceremony. We sat in our circle, and Roman concluded the ceremony by thanking the spirits for being with us.

Cynthia brought us a jar full of freshly-squeezed citrus juice, and a big bowl of delicious fruit. After fasting all day, this felt like nothing less than a generous offering from Pachamama herself. We ate and enjoyed our fruit as Roman spoke a bit more about the integration process, and how to apply the insights we gained from the medicine.

Shortly after, Elton, the Chef (who was also apprenticing to be a shaman and was once a head chef of a five-star restaurant in Italy) brought out several pots full of amazing food. We had a delicious communal feast as we shared together our individual experiences and the insights we gained. It was an amazing experience that profoundly contributed to my personal healing and spiritual growth.

As with all plant medicines, I believe they should be used with the right intention. They are powerful teachers that help us access deeper levels of our reality, and they should be respected as such. San Pedro is a mild hallucinogen, but it is still very powerful. I find it hard to explain the feeling of the medicine, as it is very subtle. In my experience, it just makes you more aware of the energy around you, and makes you more aware of things that might be too subtle for our everyday conscious awareness to notice.

In a sense, it amplifies things. For example, if I were to feel a subtle sensation of anxiety while on San Pedro, it might feel more like an intense sensation of anxiety. If I were to feel a subtle sensation of peace on San Pedro, it would feel like an intense sensation of peace. The intensification of thoughts, emotions, sensations, and energies mixed with very mild visualizations illustrates the effect that San Pedro has, at least from my experience. It can be unpleasant on the stomach, which is why it is recommended to fast while consuming it, and to also drink a lot of water. If you can learn from the discomfort instead of pushing it away, it can be one hell of a teacher.

I find it funny that no matter how much I write about a psychedelic experience, it never translates the essence of the experience itself – a reminder that words, definitions, and concepts about reality always fall short of the direct experience of reality itself. When utilized in the right way, I firmly believe that psychedelic plant medicines have a profound potential for spiritual healing and growth.

# MARINATING IN THE ESSENTIAL STEW

## Psilocybin

It's been more than six years since I participated in the Johns Hopkins Spirituality study, but it continues as the most life-changing event I've ever experienced. For those not familiar, Hopkins has been researching the effects and benefits of Psilocybin for more than a decade now. The Spirituality study, in particular, involves meditation and mantra training, counseling sessions with a guide, and two to three guided sessions mediated by Psilocybin. At the time, it all seemed straightforward enough to me. Little did I know that the content of these sessions would be so powerful that my life would change forever.

At the time of the study, I was in my early fifties, recently divorced, and relatively stable in my lifestyle and psychology. I'd worked in the field of brain injury rehabilitation for twenty years as a clinical social worker and found brain-related issues fascinating. On the spiritual front, I was raised Evangelical Christian, and even attended a major Christian college, but had taken on a loose-agnostic position over the years. Probably most importantly, I had never used a "drug" of any kind, including marijuana. This was my first foray into any mind-expanding substances. I had no idea what to expect.

The particular experimental group I was in had three sessions, each with various quantities of Psilocybin. Not surprisingly, each experience was different in both content and depth. The setting was arranged like a living room and I was invited to lie down on the couch and comfortably arrange pillows. Perhaps most importantly, for the duration of the session I was to wear an eyeshade and headphones through which played instrumental music. This ensured that the experience would be primarily internal and with distractions removed. Since there is no way I can succinctly convey all that took place in these sessions, I'll focus on several moments that were most rich and meaningful.

My "trips" were quite visual and involved journeys which led to important epiphanies about myself and the nature of all things. The descent into a Psilocybin journey for the first time is not for the faint of heart. The feeling of progressively losing control of your mind, coupled with any personal insecurities and physiological rushes made for an initial anxious experience – at least for me. The presence and wisdom of my two guides sitting beside me was critical in navigating the territory. Without them I sense I would have fought against the experience the entire way and potentially lost out on the gifts that followed.

Once immersed in the experience, I found myself being drawn into a natural amphitheater of rocks and plants. I sat down to wait on what would happen next, deeply sensing it would be meaningful. I saw a figure appear before me. It was my father who had died some forty years prior. I could feel his presence and love all around me, holding me without touch. It was his words that provided the power to press on past any fears: "Mark, you have everything you need. Don't hide, go seek," a convincing message to me, being someone who can often feel incomplete. This initial interaction would prove invaluable in preparing me for the experience that was to follow.

Shortly after my father's appearance I found myself paddling a canoe in a large lake. In a previous vision, I was shown that this lake was the container of everyone's life experience, where their rivers emptied themselves. Following the shoreline, I came across many coves until I reached one which was especially foreboding. Although fearful, I decided to explore further and paddled in. I left the boat to check out the stream that was entering the cove and when I looked back the boat was drifting away on its own. The only way was up.

I began to scramble up the stream, which was chock-full of boulders and rocks. I could feel a force of some kind drawing me to climb further and imploring me to "go to the source." The journey became more difficult, as waterfalls and large boulders blocked the way, but I found a reserve of powers and abilities, which I used to climb higher. I then found myself staring at a sixty-foot waterfall and I believed that if I could conquer it, something big would be revealed. Finding superhuman powers I was able to leap and fly to the top, only to find nothing but more streams and a path along the side to be followed. The call was still there to find the source.

I walked the path for some time, enjoying the beauty of the space, until I saw a jumble of rocks with water springing up through them. I immediately knew it as The Source. I came close and put my hands into the clear water. Never in my life had I felt something so true and beautiful. Never had I felt such an amazing peace – a "peace that passeth understanding."

It also was the most powerful place imaginable, such a rare and vital combination: peace and power. The final quality was that of compassion. The waters let me know that I was loved and accepted just as I was. This place was The Source from which all blessings flowed.

As I sat for a while and drank the water, I noticed something coming out of the brush. It was a fawn that was coming out to drink downstream. I told this to my guides who encouraged me to explore it further – to look into its eyes and discover why it was there. I was baffled for a while until it hit me… this little deer was me. It was the little deer in me that was looking for nourishment – that was looking for the healing waters of The Source. This hit me hard and I cried uncontrollably for a long time, as I could allow the little deer's pain to be felt and be held at the same time. There was a palpable sense of healing in that moment, but also a strong invitation to continue the work of healing in my everyday life. More powerfully, there was direct knowledge that this work held the key to opening locked places within me.

The third session at Hopkins was by far the most powerful and incredible. This one came with an internal guide who took on the form of a court jester, sans the outfit. A very playful, but all-knowing being who knew the territory well and was ready to show me around. "But first," he said, "we have to get someone's permission." He then reached inside me and pulled this shivering, small, fearful being out of my abdomen. The jester spoke with this being with such compassion and knowing: "You have done amazing work for Mark. I honor these beautiful walls that you created for Mark, these trenches and scaffolding that have protected him for many, many years and got him to this place. We need to make sure you're okay with taking these down so you both can fully experience the rest of this journey." The wisdom and recognition of what was needed in these initial moments still amazes me today. It was like a deeper part of me was conversing with my everyday self and delivering matter of fact truths. It would be years before I'd more fully understand this more essential self and the means of accessing it.

The experience that followed was less of a journey than an immersion into a dimension that was all-knowing, fully-compassionate, and ready to teach. Imagine a space where you are fully accepted just as you are and unencumbered by shame or doubt or fear. Where even the egoic barriers that serve to protect us are acknowledged (and even applauded to some degree), but which are no longer needed in this space. Judgment ceases. Acceptance abounds. Boundaries dissolve. What a freedom!

With my defenses lowered and full access to pure knowing and love, what followed was a complete absorption into what felt like the wisdom of the Universe. What had started as a mantra of a self-involved, "I know, I know" became the collective, "We know, we know." My knowing would be informed by a Greek chorus of ancestors, celestial teachers, and loving beings. These noetic messages were focused on simple truths. "Every move toward personal wholeness evolves the world." "Push past personal discomforts and connect with others." "Go explore the grandeur of this world." For many weeks after, my world became poetry, not prose.

A final piece of the experience still mystifies me. While marinating in the essential stew, I felt my fingers begin to move on their own, followed by my tongue, and eventually both my arms and hands joined in on the dance. They stayed in motion for several hours in what my guides said was the most beautiful dance they had ever seen. The amazing part was that I could consciously join in the dance and add my gift to whatever was happening unconsciously. I now see this as an invitation to living life... the interaction and mutual informing of the form and formless will be what creates the most meaning for us. Allowing the full integration of the two realms bears incredible fruit and may actually be what saves mankind from itself.

This account would not be complete without a discussion of the aftermath. What do you do with an experience that has rewritten your previous narrow view of the world and your place in it? How do you take the noetic download and integrate what you have seen and been given? How do I continue to "seek and not hide?"

I asked these questions of the Hopkins researchers and thankfully was provided some options. It was clear that I needed a place that could attend to both the psychological "mandates" and spiritual mysteries of the experience. Providential for me, I was drawn to a place right in Baltimore that proved to be a marvelous extension of my psychedelic experience. Inspiration Community and Consciousness School allowed me to freely explore the realms I had visited and better understand the unified relationship between psychology and spirituality.

Through experiential methods, study, and integrative breathwork, I've slowly been able to heal where healing was needed, develop deeper aspects of my being, and, in the words of Ken Wilbur, turn "states into traits." I believe this is the great invitation of psychedelics: to know there is more beyond our senses, that the truth of who we are lies within us, and that we are loved and held as we explore this vast universe, without and within.

Namaste.

*https://www.psymposia.com/magazine/my-first-psychedelic-experience-at-johns-hopkins-changed-my-life/*

# MDMA THERAPY FOR RAPE TRAUMA

## MDMA

Fifteen years ago, at the age of 15, I attended a house party where I was traumatically gang raped. At the time, I was also a virgin. I was so ashamed, humiliated, and terrified that I never spoke about it again. Until recently.

It wasn't until seven years after the sexual assault, at the age of 22, that I was ready to talk about it. I found a therapist who specialized in sexual abuse, and in addition to one-on-one therapy I entered group therapy for sexually abused women. After two years of counseling and group therapy, I assumed that, since I had finally come to a place where I could at least talk about my rape, I was "healed," not really knowing what being healed looked like.

Throughout the years, I continued to struggle with intimacy and trust, never correlating these deep issues to my rape. Regardless of my ability to acknowledge the trauma, it was always difficult to talk about. Anytime it would come up in conversation, I felt my sympathetic nervous system getting activated through heart palpitations and the sense of "fight, flight, or freeze," along with feelings of shame and embarrassment. The truth was I was far from healed.

Fast forward to the age of 30. Through a random conversation unrelated to my rape, I was triggered and re-experienced the effects of my sexual assault. For two weeks I such as nightmares and random panic attacks. During the panic attacks, which sometimes lasted as long as twenty to thirty minutes, I had a strange feeling of not being safe. It was confusing and unusual. I realized I was resurfacing the familiar feeling of "fear of death" that I had experienced during my rape.

I had been seeing a therapist for about a year, so I discussed this new trigger with him. We decided MDMA was an appropriate therapy to explore in order to release the trauma. We had done two MDMA sessions before to help with childhood pain, so I was familiar. I now realize that my rape was responsible for most of the other trauma and current pain in my life. It was the major source of my pain.

The day before our scheduled MDMA session, I had a meltdown. I was terrified of feeling the pain surrounding my rape and afraid that I would be re-traumatized given the PTSD I experienced when it first triggered. I almost cancelled the session.

The morning of my MDMA session – and before I ingested the medicine – I had nonstop diarrhea, sweaty palms, heart palpitations, and cottonmouth. I was unbelievably terrified to face it. I'm sharing this to provide insight on how much trauma I had stored inside my body, even fifteen years later.

My friend drove me to meet my therapist at 8:45 a.m. and it took forty-five minutes for the medicine to kick in.

When I met my therapist at his office, I was terrified and holding back a panic attack. I could hardly speak; my voice was shaky and my heart was pounding full blast. I lied on the couch curled into a ball while he kept trying to help me ground myself by saying, "Why don't you go into the pain and do exactly what your body wants you to do?"

At 9:30 a.m. I ingested another 50 mg of MDMA, which we previously discussed as a way to prolong the peak of the medicine and allow more time for therapeutic work. My severe anxiety continued for an hour and a half into the session – well after the MDMA took effect. Usually after it kicks in I feel good, open, and ready to share.

This experience of severe anxiety was unusual for me. My therapist kept trying to get me to describe the pain I was feeling as I laid, now curled in a ball on the floor. I kept fidgeting; no matter what position I was in I was horribly uncomfortable. I just wanted to hide from the severe pain I was feeling in my chest.

Finally, I sat up and asked my therapist to bring me back to the trauma through an "elevator" meditation we had done in the past. I came to do this work and was damned if my fears were going to get the best of me.

He had me visualize stepping into the elevator with him and we hit the fifteenth floor – to represent my age at the time of the trauma. The elevator door opened and he said, "You are at a party. Tell me what you see." I shouted in panic, "Don't leave me!" He replied, "I'm right here in the elevator waiting for you and not going anywhere." I walked into the party and began recalling exactly what I remembered.

After all these years I have never been able to remember

exactly what happened that night. It was always very foggy. While on MDMA, I was able to recall most of the night. My visual memory was sporadic; I didn't always have an image to match the words coming out of my mouth because I believe the shock blocked it out, but my mouth was confidently telling a story I had never heard before. I remembered conversations, specific faces, and even feelings that occurred for me throughout the night. I've read MDMA allows memories to resurface since it affects the amygdala.

We got to the actual rape and my body started playing out the incident. I started screaming in the office, "No, please, stop!! Someone is hitting me! Someone else is also in the room! They are just watching! I'm terrified! No one is helping! NO ONE IS HELPING!!"

I felt a burning in my chest. It was cold and at the same time felt like heartburn. I felt actual pain of pure terror, which I now realize was the fear of death. I realized that the night I was raped, I thought they were going to kill me. I recognized that my reaction the day before and the morning of this session was because the trauma was surfacing. I've carried around this terror in my body for fifteen years.

As I started shouting, "NO ONE IS HELPING!!" my inner thighs began to tremble, where in my meditation I was being penetrated. Then my legs, chest, and whole body were shaking viciously. Scared, I shouted to my therapist, "What's happening?!" He calmly reassured me, "It's okay. Your body is just releasing some trauma." I must have shaken for a whole five minutes. I imagine I looked like a fish out of water. The shaking eventually slowed and I took a bunch of big deep breaths.

I turned to him and said, "Wow, what was that?!" His reassuring smile told me that he had seen this before. It's obvious that I was releasing shock and deeply stored trauma. Many victims of physical trauma report that painful memories are stored in the body and it's our body's natural reaction to shake out the trauma. However, due to shame and embarrassment, we push our feelings/shaking back down. Today you can find Trauma Release Exercises where people shake their bodies in an attempt to release the trauma.

After the first shaking episode, we went back into the meditation. I continued to role-play the traumatic event. The shaking continued each time I approached another feeling that I had stuffed deep inside. Just after the rape reenactment finished, I felt intense humiliation. I remembered that after I had been raped I was left lying on the bed, alone, naked, and in shock. My friend, who later found me at the party, was trying to talk to me, but I couldn't respond. She thought I was unconscious, but really, I was in shock and couldn't speak.

I began to feel the same exact humiliation that I had felt fifteen years earlier. To finally be in touch with that pain again was phenomenal. I wanted to hide from the feeling. It was literally so painful in my chest. As I said out loud, "Ugggghhh the humiliation, it hurts! Humiliation!" My body began to compulsively shake again and I shook out all of the humiliation.

I then began reenacting how I felt the day after the rape. The morning after, I remember seeing blood between my legs and a little on my shirt from my bloody nose. I also had a black

207

eye for about a week. I remembered lying in my bed at home, in shock, feeling so much shame. I felt dirty and unlovable and I didn't think anyone would ever want me. I was now no longer a virgin.

I said to my therapist, "I feel deflated," and laid on the floor of his office and reenacted feeling deflated. Just then I felt a pulsation of deep shame and again – a cold yet burning pain in my chest. Like clockwork, my body began to shake out the shame. With each shake I could feel this break of energy. I literally felt lighter.

Thanks to the MDMA, I was no longer shaming myself. After each shake, I would tell myself that the men who raped me should be humiliated, not me. I am so lovable and have so much to offer. I let myself know that today I had nothing to fear and could let go of my paranoia surrounding close relationships. These were all things I needed to hear after the rape happened and finally I was able to offer it to myself. It's one thing for a therapist to tell you that you have nothing to fear, but it's another to believe it and hear it come from yourself. I could feel I was now at the peak of the MDMA experience.

Next, I moved onto rage. I said, "I feel so used! They used me!!" I grabbed a pillow and screamed into it at the top of my lungs. Never in my life did I think it was possible to get angry and scream while on MDMA. We had previously discussed in therapy that "being used" was a trigger for me and anytime I felt used in my day-to-day life I experienced intense rage. It was such a huge release to finally let go of that deep anger, the source of that trigger, which had affected me for YEARS. Finally, I understood how much baggage I had been carrying and finally, I was removing it. With the help of MDMA, I was able to see my own worth and confront my shame with kindness.

Unknowingly, there was one more thing I needed to reenact to receive peace from this traumatic story. I needed and yearned for reassurance from my father that I was a lovable person, that he wasn't disgusted or disappointed with me, and that he loved me. Not receiving this, as my father never talked to me about my rape, greatly affected how I learned to cope. To this day, that affects my relationship with him. Having worked with my therapist for a year, at times, I looked to him as a father figure.

When I came down from the MDMA, I asked him for a hug and mentioned that I felt like a disgusting person for what happened to me. He held me, rubbed my back as a father would to their child and reassured me that I am not disgusting and that I am a good person. While some professionals may see this as crossing boundaries, we both had healthy boundaries and trust for each other that had built over the course of the year. This transference was imperative for me to release the last piece of trauma that had haunted me for years – that my father didn't love me.

I sat back down on the couch and felt profound, absolute bliss in my chest after a morning of intense pain. It felt like I had multiple knots inside my chest that had finally been untangled. I was also able to breathe easier and deeper. I was feeling so overwhelmed with love for myself, a feeling I had not experienced before. Instead, I usually experienced a recorded tape of self-hatred that had been on repeat for fifteen fucking years – that it was my fault, that I was unlovable, that I should be ashamed, and that I'm damaged goods. Finally, I was free from it.

Without MDMA, I don't think I could have faced those terrible and physically painful feelings. My body literally would not allow me to go there during regular talk therapy. My fear response would sound off before I could reach inside the feeling.

We usually plan our MDMA sessions to be five hours; however, I felt done with all the work I needed to do and recovered from the session in just four hours. Typically, the MDMA will last for three hours and I will slowly come down over the next two hours. For the first time, I felt clear and sober in a shorter amount of time.

At 1 p.m. my friend came and picked me up and stayed the afternoon with me while I napped. I felt exhausted from all of the exertion of energy. Companionship following an MDMA session is essential to feeling safe and supported while continuing to come down off the medicine. I'm never fully sober until about four hours after the session ends.

Later that evening, I noticed that my chronic shoulder, neck, and back pain that I've had for years were completely gone. For years I have always ached. I figured it was because I sat at a computer all day, but now I realize that it was stored trauma in my body causing knots in my muscles. I also slept a solid nine hours the night of the session, which was rare for me. For months leading up to this session, I would wake up throughout the night with anxiety. I woke up the next day feeling content and at peace – something I hadn't felt in a while.

One of the most profound effects was my ability to breathe deeper in my chest. Today, four months later, the pain in my neck and shoulders is still gone. I can also tell my rape story without feeling heart palpitations or being triggered.

I am incredibly grateful for a therapist who was willing to look beyond the restrictions placed on MDMA and grant me the healing I so desperately needed. It pains me that therapists are forced to risk their licenses while using this incredible tool. So many other people are carrying around their trauma and may continue to for the rest of their lives if MDMA-assisted psychotherapy is not made available to them.

I lived with this pain for fifteen years. FIFTEEN FUCKING YEARS! It is one of my greatest hopes that other people with intense, stored trauma will be able to access this same kind of healing. I urge therapists and people suffering from trauma and PTSD to educate themselves on the benefits of MDMA therapy.

*https://www.psymposia.com/magazine/mdma-assisted-psychotherapy-for-rape-trauma/*

# A RED MARBLE SKY

## Psilocybin

It was a few years ago in February when my first excursion into the spiritual realm with magic mushrooms commenced. I was curious to discover the unknown entities that lived among us in different states, within our dreams, within our own subconscious, and in the metaphysical realm of spiritual enlightenment. I had done my research. I read books on the subject and inquired about their effects on the mind and body with several friends of mine. Their response was unanimous; they all said it was wild and amazing, beautiful and transformative. I knew at that moment that whatever apprehension I was feeling that may have prevented me from going through with my plans was quickly evaporating. This was the time, and now was the hour.

I nearly laughed out loud when I saw Psilocybin mushrooms for the first time in my life. I opened the bag and took a big whiff. It smelled pungent. I knew immediately that the worse the odor was, the stronger the trip would be. I was obsessing over what my experience would be, what I would see and hear, and how my senses would be greatly heightened, improved, and sharpened to the best of their ability.

We stopped for dinner and ate like kings. I wanted to have a full stomach before my trip. We went back to my house and got everything ready. I prepared the Blu-ray player and connected it with my TV. I had Stanley Kubrick's *2001: A*

*Space Odyssey* in my hands. I figured if we were to watch a movie it was going to be this one, especially with something like mushrooms. It was time to start this party off with a bang!

I stared at the opened bag in fascination. Inside were large plump stems with giant caps on top, and I thought to myself how they packed a wallop inside. There were unexplored territories inside of them, uncharted universes within universes, places we didn't have the faintest understanding of, things we'd only been acquainted with in our dreams. I held the first mushroom stem to my nose and inhaled its odor. I threw it in my mouth, sucked out the juice inside, and chewed it. It tasted horrendous, but as I digested it I knew there was no turning back.

It took a good solid hour for it to really kick in and take effect, but as it did I felt lighter, calmer, happier, and more in harmony with the world around me. A wave of euphoria lifted me up and kept me elevated. It was tremendous to feel how the mushrooms amplified my outlook on life. It was a power like I'd never seen before and a doorway that had been kicked the fuck down.

A half hour further into my trip, the party started getting rowdy. It was spellbinding, and while I watched 2001 it was clear to me that it wasn't just me that was in league with the spiritual realm, but everyone in my life too. Memories came flooding back to me at once and everything that I had endured and experienced and remembered from childhood revealed itself in the thaw. Memories of being young and free, going over my grandmother's house which was just like a beautiful mansion, using the pool, enjoying the sunlight, taking advantage of everything that life had to offer, family, inner happiness, and friendship. I remember having the best times over there, feeling content and not worrying what tomorrow would bring, not concerning myself with bills, or my job, or a new car, or the new iPhone, or an apartment – the really futile pointless evils which we are burdened with every day in our society were not in my life at that point.

That's what can mushrooms do. They can allow us to see the big picture and give us the chance to see the entire galaxy instead of just counting the stars. It was consuming and it was revelatory.

I saw colors morph into each other and I heard sounds that were alien, but fascinating too. I saw the floor in my living room breathe to life. The faces of the people in the movie disappeared and reappeared simultaneously, almost as if they were being reconstructed in my brain. It was surreal! The movie was like an echo of the mushrooms themselves and what was happening inside of me. The blast of sound, color, music, and of course the space stations, the spaceships themselves, the characters, the movement, the composition, the one-point perspective which is used consistently by Kubrick in all of his films, all of it was a reflection of the soul. This was life everlasting. This was a meditation on mankind. This film was life itself, from our conception into the Universe to our death and back again, reincarnated, recalibrated, wiser, better.

When I saw the character Dave slip down a wormhole in space I gasped out loud, because it wasn't just happening to him, it was happening to me as well. I was passing from one world into another, glancing past the horizon into a higher truth. I was being reborn.

I paused the movie, and as I went downstairs to get some beer, I recall having the feeling that I could fly down to the basement. I felt so light and so unencumbered by the pressures and stress of everyday reality; it was almost as if an invisible force was pulling me toward my destination.

As these euphoric feelings came over me, my friend shouted down to ask me to bring up some water. I nearly shit my pants because my house felt even quieter than usual, and being in the basement wasn't exactly heaven. When I was in the basement, I had the distinct feeling that I was underground in some secret mansion in the hills. It all felt so big and massive and expanded my cerebral cortex enormously, so everything around me was like an infinite hallway. Spaces moved and stretched, yet stayed the same. Colors changed like a chameleon blending in with the corridors of the mind. It was like a spiritual rebirth, a change that was rapidly coming to fruition inside me. It made me question the old adage "the Universe is in the palm of your hand" when really, the palm of your hand is the Universe!

I went back upstairs and my friend and I went outside into the giant blizzard. To my amazement, everything around me – the trees, the sky, the air, the stars, and the moon – appeared to be made of glass; sheer, clear, smooth glass. I held my hand against the air and felt as if I could easily shatter the glass to discover what was behind all this beauty.

We whipped out the bowl packed with weed and lit up. The smoke lingered in the air like a cloud of rain and it was so loaded with flavor I started coughing in the still February night. I stopped and sat there overlooking the winter storm, weeping at the beauty of the early morning darkness. The trees outside of my house looked like dark skeletons, their long branches stretching endlessly into the night sky. The blizzard reminded me of a friendly tornado. It didn't devour everything in its path, but instead it softened it. It felt like something out of a movie.

I thought to myself how quiet my neighborhood was and how peaceful and serene it was. It was beautiful. It was so desolate you could hear your own heartbeat. It felt as if we were the only two people left on Earth. Two friends in a spiritual conference with an invisible presence. I was right where I was meant to be, under the winter skies of a blizzard, an astonishing event indeed.

We sat out there for another ten minutes before we realized it was time to go in and warm up by the fire. I switched the fireplace on and as the flames inside the electric fireplace blazed up so did I. I hit the bowl once more and that's when I really started seeing beyond the horizon.

My friend and I sat in the dark in the TV room. As I shut the TV off, I just listened to the silence. The clear undisturbed sound of quiet. The whisper of the world I had created around me. Nearly in a meditative state of consciousness, the wind outside filled my ears like a classical symphony. I couldn't pull myself away from glancing out the window of my living room at the wind howling in the distance. It resembled the sound the tornado made in The Wizard of Oz.

My house itself felt bigger to me. My spatial awareness was

was heightened enormously. The walls seemed to move further and further away from me and the doors and stairs were almost too huge for a house to contain. It was the painting of the mushrooms laid bare, the truth behind the lie, and the reality inside the illusion. *2001: A Space Odyssey* blasted me into the spiritual netherworld of higher consciousness, and Cube was the navigation around that spiritual world and the different paths of enlightenment.

An important word comes to mind any time I take psychedelics: echoes. Echoes of sound, laughter, life, and dreams replay in the mind like a stream of consciousness. It all reveals itself; the colors and mood of a cold winter night or the bright sunshine of a cloudless summer afternoon. All of it comes back like a heavy boomerang. Echoes of great vacations, echoes of a broken heart, echoes of a great night out for your birthday, all the good and all of the bad and the cohesion of the two. They don't call these babies magic mushrooms for nothing!

The slow come down from the mushrooms was beginning to commence. It was mystical and it was over in the blink of an eye. Just like that, it comes, you fall in love, and then it's gone and you're back in the real world. Back in the perceived reality of life. And you smile. But it's a paradox, isn't it? You're happy to be back, but you also wonder what else there is beyond the rainbow to see and experience. I'm not too sure… there's something though.

My friend and I passed out in the living room, exhausted after some rather large energy expenditure, slipping into the outer banks of our minds, the unrelenting fire. We had a blast careening through the Universe, feeling connected with nature, the snowstorm, and a dark red marble sky. It was intense, it was potent, and it was exhilarating. It made me smile, laugh, cry, and shout. It made me happy with where I was and with what I had. The way Dorothy always had the power to go back to Kansas; we as a species also have the power within us to change our world.

I woke up and the sky was a blinding orb of sunlight, a wintery blast of cold covered everything. The sky was white and the mushrooms left a happy surprise, a euphoric high even when my trip was done. It was a celebration for my mind, and life is a celebration. "So, what did you think?" my friend asked as he helped himself to some water. "That was fucking amazing," I responded. "What's next dude?"

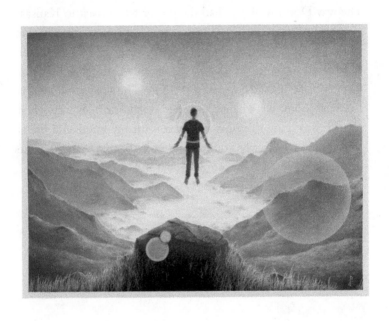

# THE NEW BIRTH

## LSD

It was well known to my close circle of friends that I had always been interested in a psychedelic experience. I had already dabbled with MDMA and the feelings of oneness I felt while under the influence of MDMA were AMAZING! I knew that the feeling could be intense with psychedelics and I was ready to have an out of this world experience. I did not think it could be life changing like Ayahuasca, Peyote or DMT. I did however think that I would go into an imaginary cartoon world or a world of gibberish.

So here I was, 8:09 p.m. to be exact, and I dropped my very first LSD tab. I was way too pumped now and everyone could see it on my face. But here it was, the part I hated the most: waiting for it to hit. I waited and waited, tried to be distracted, but then almost two hours had passed. I could not believe it. Substances usually hit me within twenty minutes of me taking them. So, my friends, being the best friends they are to me, said that it was time to eat the mushrooms.

I started to wrap my mushrooms in my favorite candy, Fruit by the Foot and ate them. Twenty minutes had passed and I started to get the giggles; colors were driving around my living room floor and it began.

I was stuck. I sounded like a broken record. On repeat, I kept saying the same things over and over. "Hi, who are you?"

and "Hello, are you there?" were just a couple of phrases that I kept repeating over and over every time I made eye contact with someone. I started to question why this was happening. My friends would tell me that I was high. I couldn't believe that I was high – high off of what? What was LSD? Why would I have disoriented myself this way on purpose? I could not make sense of anything. As this was happening I kept falling asleep about every ten minutes. I would get extremely sleepy, close my eyes, and then wake up as if I had never fallen asleep and start in with my same questions. It was a cycle that felt like days, but it had only been about two hours.

As I started to gain more control and slowly started to get unstuck, I was becoming less disoriented. Still sleepy, I buried my face into my husband's chest. Before this exact moment, I had no memories of the moments in between the broken record cycle. Therefore, this was my first intense moment of my trip.

As I buried my face into his chest, I closed my eyes. It felt so warm. His heartbeat was so peaceful. Suddenly I had turned into a baby in the womb. I was in my womb. I was my baby. I was my two-year-old son! Sucking on my thumb, the warmth consumed me and I felt every ounce of love in the Universe. I do not know how to better explain what all the love in the world would feel like, but that is exactly what I felt. It was the happiest feeling I have ever felt. I had no idea that this much love existed or that one could feel this much love at once! It was so peaceful.

As I lifted my head and opened my eyes, the lights were shining in my face and a team of nurses were surrounding me. I felt the love of those nurses as they fought hard to breathe for me and keep me alive. They did not know me; I was a newborn baby. How could they love me so much? How could they fight for my life so hard? I broke into tears. Emotions vacillated between happiness and sadness. I had always felt appreciation for those nurses who were in the delivery room with us during my son's birth, but experiencing that moment through him was life changing.

After I burst into tears my thoughts started pouring in. Why am I so short tempered with my baby? Why do I have so much resentment? How is it his fault? Why is he paying the price of my emotions? I love him! I know I do, but how could it be so easy for me to be so disconnected from him? My marriage was very rocky when I found out that I was expecting him and I knew that was the reason for the feelings of resentment I had during and after my pregnancy. This experience brought me to my knees. I started to question all the ugliness I had inside. I started to question everything about me, about others, and about our thoughts.

As I started to be more aware of where I was, I "realized" that I had died and I was in the afterlife. The afterlife was a huge disappointment. It was my living room. I couldn't believe that after all that living, this is where I would end up – my living room. It was an infinite nothingness. I was shocked! I couldn't believe that the life I had lived was made up in my own mind. No one existed and I had made everyone up. I started asking my husband where everyone was. Where were my boys? Where was my mom? I told him that I remembered giving birth. Why did they not exist? Vivid memories of the events that happened that day before the LSD flooded my mind – vivid memories of close friends and people that I loved. They felt so real, but in my mind, it was all made up. Nothing. No one existed.

From this point forward I spent the rest of my trip crying, devastated with the nothingness that surrounded me. My circle of friends was physically there, but it didn't feel like it at all. I no longer wanted that luxury car because it didn't matter. It felt as if I had something better than that. I no longer wanted any of these luxuries that we all work so hard to have because it felt as if I possessed them all. Feeling as if I had everything I could possibly ever want, but knowing I did not have any of it made me want something so much more meaningful. What I wanted most was to change my ways. Change the way I think, the way I act, and the things I say. I wanted to radiate the love I felt and shine as bright as the sun! Those things held so much more value than any materialistic thing I could ever want here on Earth.

Heartbroken at who I was and what I had become, it was now 5 a.m. and I had a blank stare almost as if I was empty; as if my soul had left me. Nothingness. But then I felt a shift inside of me and felt more aware as the minutes continued to pass. Little by little, I felt in full control. I could feel myself coming back. In the background, I heard *Feeling Good* remixed by Bassnectar. "It's a new dawn, it's a new day, it's a new life for me and I'm feeling good…" and I cried tears of joy. I was alive! I was back! Everything was the way I had left it. It was not a dream It was all so real, but it also wasn't. I can't find the right words to explain what I felt in that moment as my song played, but wow, I got a second chance at a few things I was not okay with and that is priceless.

# DITCHING MY CRUTCHES & SCALING MOUNTAINS

## LSD

All around me was the undeniable majesty of Joshua Tree. I'd thought I'd be floored by the alien tree structures, since that's what the national park is named after, but I had not expected the gorgeous prehistoric-feeling rock formations stacking into the sky.

All this around me, and I was on crutches, my hip a mess. I had come to Joshua Tree to celebrate New Year's Eve by tripping with nine of my best friends. We'd scoped the expansive park and found the place we wanted to use as our base camp for the day's adventures.

We had all our provisions set up – blankets to deal with the cold we knew would come with the desert dusk, a tab of LSD for each of us, snacks for those who could eat while tripping, and our mascot Spartacus, a baby eagle stuffed animal who would watch over our stuff while we were off exploring. He's very astute with those eagle eyes. And I, of course, had my crutches. I couldn't part with them without extreme hip pain.

Let me interrupt myself to say that crutches are by no means the worst thing to happen to an adventuring person, or any person really. My injury had only been going on for a couple months, whereas some people live with differently abled bodies for their entire lives and are able to conquer mountains far greater than the piles of rocks in Joshua Tree National Park. But crutches and leg injuries alike are a hindrance, to say the least, to off-roading – particularly to someone unpracticed in navigating uneven terrain with crutches. I was worried about my ability to keep up with my more able-bodied friends during our trip, but tried not to let it faze me.

So there we were, provisions all around us, bundled in coats against the cold. We passed out the tabs of LSD, we toasted, and we dropped. And then we waited.

We reminded ourselves of the cardinal rules of tripping: gravity is real, drugs are not food, beer is not water. Cars are real. To which we added, for the particularities of our setting: everything is sharp. If you've ever been to Joshua Tree, you'll know that all the plants out there are pretty much of the cactus variety and the rocks are also very pointy.

Already before the LSD kicked in, one of our party sat on a cactus, "Unintentionally," she explained as we took turns picking nearly invisible cactus needles out of her butt. As if anyone would wittingly opt for that unpleasant experience.

And then suddenly, up we went. First a glimmer and that familiar vibrate-y feeling in our stomachs and extremities, and then the rocks started to shimmer and melt into giant embracing gorillas. We sat there, perched on the rocks, as we acclimated to our new reality. And then, one by one, my friends peeled off to explore.

I sat on a rock by myself, trying to remember why I wasn't moving with the rest. There was some reason, but I just couldn't remember it. Oh right, my hip was messed up and I'd been hobbling around for weeks in a considerable amount of shooting pain from my right hip to my knee. But there were my friends, scaling cliffs, lizarding around in the sunshine. I wanted to join in! I stood up, gingerly putting my weight on my right leg. And… nothing. No pain. No tenderness. I was invincible.

Speaking about this moment later, my partner said it was such a shocking transformation that he didn't believe it. One moment I was on crutches, and the next I was bouldering about. But in retrospect, I'm not surprised. The brain is a powerful meaning-maker.

And since that trip, I've learned a lot about how pain works. Pain actually isn't as direct a response as "body part gets injured, then you feel pain." What actually happens is that your brain is receiving and reading constant nerve signals from every part of your body, no matter how small, and deciding whether those signals indicate danger. If your brain assesses sufficient danger, then it causes you to feel pain so that you stop doing whatever it is that is making you feel that way and instead spend your energy taking care of your parts. The problem with longer-term (also called chronic) pain is that the cause of the danger response can actually have gone away, but your brain can remain stuck on it and keep your body in an active state of pain as a result.

So what happened with my miracle leg healing? My hypothesis is that my hip had actually gotten better more or less, with my two plus months of crutching and otherwise being gentle with it. Now it needed to be used to build back up muscle, but my brain was still afraid.

Those of us who have personal experience with psychedelics

know that part of a hallucinogenic experience is the sloughing off of deeply embedded fears. Researchers are currently revitalizing rigorous research into this phenomenon, as most recently and comprehensively reported in *The Trip Treatment* by Michael Pollan. I was afraid to hurt my hip again, and so I treated it too kindly. I needed to run and be free, and LSD helped me do that.

*https://www.psymposia.com/magazine/how-lsd-helped-me-ditch-my-crutches-and-scale-mountains/*

# AWAKENING TO THE INFINITE

## Ayahuasca

I was fortunate enough to spend thirty-three days in an off-grid community in a very sacred place where the Amazon rainforest meets the Andes Mountains in Peru. It was an unforgettable experience that I am very grateful for. On this journey, I was studying Permaculture, Shamanism, and the Ancestral wisdom traditions of the Indigenous Amazonian and Andean people. I participated in various ceremonies, from shamanic breathwork to San Pedro cactus, to Coca circles, and ceremonial Cacao. However, one of the most healing ceremonies of all was the Ayahuasca ceremony.

I had always been curious what the Ayahuasca experience would be like, and I also knew that it would be helpful for my personal healing and spiritual growth, so I was very open to taking the medicine when the opportunity was presented to me. On the day of the Ayahuasca ceremony, we began with an amazing lecture about the cultural traditions of Ayahuasca and its history, purpose, and healing power. Afterwards we had a few hours to reflect and prepare. I decided to bathe in the river and then began reading a beautiful book titled *Celebrating Silence*.

I read about a hundred pages until I heard the sound of the Ram's horn being blown, signifying that it was time to gather for the ceremony. We all gathered in our spots, and Roman, our shaman, briefly discussed the practical tips and general advice for drinking Ayahuasca. Then, he sang a song to call in the Spirits so that they could be present with us and protect us through the ceremony.

The temple was very dark – being lit only by three candles in the center of the space. Roman passed an Ayahuasca vine to his right, and the person who received the vine held it to their forehead and began stating their intention. Stating your intention for using the medicine is a powerful tradition, and it helps to clarify why you are taking the medicine, and what you hope the medicine will be able to help you with.

When the vine was passed to me, I held it to my forehead and began speaking, "My intention is to become more aware of my true self, to acknowledge the illusions that are preventing me from realizing my true self, and to let go of these illusions so that I may be free. Please help me see all that I have been hiding from myself." I passed the vine along, and sat in silence. I dwelled in this calm meditative space as I listened to the intentions of the others in the group.

Once our intentions were stated, the first person to Roman's right got up and kneeled before him. Roman stared at him for a moment, and then filled up a wooden cup with the Ayahuasca brew. "Salud," said the man. "Salud," we mirrored back, as he tilted his head back and drank the medicine.

I watched as each person went to take their drink, and eventually it was my turn. I approached Roman and kneeled before him as he poured my cup and blessed it. He then handed it to me. "Salud," I said, as the group mirrored back. I downed the medicine like a shot of alcohol. It was bitter, sweet, tangy, and had an Earthy, wood-like taste to it. It was an interesting taste and it was very strong. I found it to be neither enjoyable, nor disgusting, but the consistency was rather thick.

I went back to my spot and sat in meditation, trying to be very present with the medicine as it made its way through my body. After each person took their shot, one of the community members got up and blew out all the candles. It was pitch black. I sat there and really tried to feel the medicine inside of me. It was upsetting my stomach but the discomfort wasn't too severe.

About twenty minutes had passed and still there was nothing unusual besides the stomach discomfort. I remember thinking that it probably wouldn't be too intense. Sure enough, almost immediately after that thought entered my mind, I heard someone vomiting in the darkness nearby.

Shortly after, I felt the effects of the medicine coming on. There was no "come up" or gradual increase in the effect, but rather a bunch of intense and powerful sensations seemed to arise altogether out of nowhere. It felt as if it was coming from above my body and descending into my field of vision.

I must mention ahead of time that the whole experience is truly unexplainable. Limited words do almost nothing to explain the vastness and complexity of the Ayahuasca experience. I will do my best to explain it, but really, the medicine opens you up to a reality that is beyond words, beyond description, and beyond anything we are familiar with in our typical daily lives. It opens you up to the multidimensional continuum in which everything is happening all together at once, and short sequences of linear words are simply insufficient in translating the experience. I mention this because what I am about to explain sounds very strange, but it is the best possible way that I can describe what was happening.

I saw and felt a vivid array of vibrational patterns slowly sinking toward me. The patterns were a mix of purple, green, yellow, and black, and in the patterns were two arms, also descending toward me. The arms seemed to be a part of the pattern, but were also distinct from it. They gradually approached my head as they swayed back and forth in a snake-like manner. Unexpectedly, I felt a very nurturing and mother-like energy coming from the arms, and felt that I could trust them.

The arms wrapped around, then entered into my body as if to work on my body from the inside. The sensations were so sudden, so powerful, so overwhelming, and intense that I instantly regretted taking the medicine. However, I knew that I could not un-drink the medicine, and I had to surrender to the experience. I decided to allow the medicine to do its work, as I sat in my witnessing awareness and watched whatever it was that was happening to me.

As soon as I surrendered fully, before me was a vast dance of vibrational energy. My awareness zoomed out from my regular field of vision, and as it did, my ego, body, and mind seemed to dissolve completely in this awareness. I realized that my ego or the idea of "me" was just a story that I maintained – a dream – and it had no reality other than the reality that I gave to it. Not only that, but it was such a small bubble of existence that had imprisoned me and confined me from the greater reality of my being.

Well, that small bubble of ego had popped. I saw beyond it. I saw life in its totality. I was the eternal Self, the Consciousness of God witnessing the dance of energy, with each energy being existing as a form that this formless Consciousness inhabited. I realized that my life story wasn't my story, just a story – one that was not real, but one that I just told myself and clung to for comfort. I realized deeply that my existence was my responsibility, that my life was a piece of art that was given to the divine – the greater organism that I was a part of. I felt that my purpose was to just be myself and to give back to the all, but in a way that was my own unique creative expression.

During all of these realizations, Roman and his wife Cynthia were singing sacred songs called Icaros, playing drums, rattles, and flutes, holding space for the ceremony, and maintaining the collective energy. I truly admired their strength and the work that they did. It was such a beautiful ceremony, and I felt that I was just an open and empty awareness witnessing this divine play of music, color, and vibration.

There was so much energy before me. I could see the frequency waves being emitted from the various things around me – the musical instruments, the people in the room, the crickets and birds outside the temple, the celestial spirits. Everything appeared to be giving off a wave of vibration, and all of these vibratory emissions were just dancing together in a field of spacial awareness.

I stepped outside of my illusion, into the truth of life. That is the best that I can do to put this beautiful and indescribable experience into words. It was a night full of love, awe, euphoria, peace, freedom, clarity, laughter, joy, beauty, and mystery, and I will never forget it.

I saw myself die and felt what was beyond. I have no doubt that after death, my soul lives on, and that I am always loved by my divine mother and father. I have trust in the Universe now, and I can finally relax. I am free.

# UNPLUGGING FROM THE MATRIX

## LSD

Firefly and I, both looking for crystal clear clarity from the Universe for our future paths, decided to close out the year with psychedelic journeying at Intention, a winter festival. We created a sacred space, set our intentions and sealed them by placing a crystal between our held hands and asking for pure white light and only the highest powers to surround us, support us, and guide us. We took our LSD tabs and the instant visual I was given was of children lined up to receive communion wafers from a priest.

We decided to go to the Loving Room next door to us, which had now been turned into a rave scene with pumping music. After dancing for a bit, we ended up at the front of the room by the altar and began playing with the crystals. I picked up a massive clear quartz crystal, my favorite type of crystal, and felt the music and the energy pulsing through and from it. We put our crystals to our foreheads and the energy coming off them was immense and pulsed from my third eye to his. We played around with the crystals a bit and checked out the sacred geometry pictures which now had considerable depth to them. You could get lost in them. We danced some more and then settled in the back of the room lying down amongst a pile of cushions.

We were transported into a euphoric state almost instantly. I could feel a simple touch on the arm through my entire being, touch amplified to the extreme. I turned to Firefly, "We just hit the jackpot. We were all prepared for an intense journey," and all we can hear is, "You are in perfect alignment. Your intuition separately and together is flawless. You are shown things and you listen even though nothing makes sense to you according to logic. You dig, and unearth who you really are. You do the work. Now it's time to have fun kids."

We were having the most intense experience, similar to MDMA, but so much richer and with incredible depth. It was a feeling of being completely enveloped and embraced in love, with touch being a completely transcendent experience. We were laughing, just rolling and fully enjoying the ride. We changed from flying through the Universe at warp speed, to jumping off and through galaxies to diving from one solar system to the next and into infinity, an immensity totally consuming, and then sometimes we would be the same galaxy sharing the same experience and sometimes we would merge, mesh and cross over each other all simultaneously. I have never seen or experienced my divinity so clearly. After all these months of typing my password "limitless" daily, trying to taste it, I finally fully felt it and knew in that moment I would never question it again.

Our journey was rudely interrupted by a phone call regarding a "family emergency." Our groggy bodies rose to deal with the situation. Our friend Zoe escorted us back to the cabin and back to another reality. A phone call was made and an angry hateful voice spewed venom on the other side. Something about a Wi-Fi password, not even close to an emergency. What a relief. And then I felt an instant acknowledgement of the situation Firefly was in. A controller was feeling threatened. Familiar with that, I understood and was reminded that people only operate from their level of consciousness and hurt people hurt people. All I could do was feel the chaos of feelings on the other end of the phone. The whole time, I was whispering in Firefly's ear, "Love, love, love." This was drilled into me from my experience, when I asked the Universe, "What do I do?" the answer always came back as love. No matter what comes back at you, always love.

The conversation ended and we laid down in bed. Moments later there was a shift. Everywhere my mind went, there was a mirror showing me what I thought was real wasn't and things turned into what can only be described as a personal hell. My mind was preying on every weakness and block, challenging and limiting my beliefs, which all boiled down to trust and surrender. My rock and grounding Firefly morphed into the devil, or a version of him, and I was shown a past life that screamed at me that I was in danger from him. It was the ultimate final exam in trust and surrender, but this time I heard, "Love. Love is the answer. You know this."

I started throwing love left and right chanting "love, love, love" and the more love I threw around the more the confusion and chaos dissipated. Firefly returned back to himself and all the challenges, blocks, limiting beliefs and past traumas evaporated like someone in a video game just came in with an AK-47 and annihilated them. I was shown why we are really here on Earth and remembered part of that from Freezer Burn, a summer festival I journeyed at, but this time it was much clearer. Every single interaction with any other person or situation has to do with soul development, which is why it is so important to spread love everywhere we go. By showing kindness, taking the time to smile and comment on the cashier's necklace, opening doors, and letting people into our lane when driving, we are showing their souls the right direction – the direction away from the chaos and the dark and back into the light where they belong. It may seem like nothing, but that soul will remember and will keep following, if not the person, then the feeling of love and light that the soul delivered to them, until eventually it finds its own path out of the dark.

Our souls have many lessons to learn from overcoming guilt, forgiveness, betrayal, heartache, death, and loss to name a few. Our soul development requires us to learn these lessons; however, it would be too much to learn them all in one lifetime, so we choose one or two lessons to learn during each lifetime. Then when we die/transition, we have a chance to renegotiate and come back as a different physical being to learn more soul lessons or be a guide from above for a bit.

I woke up hours later. My bladder was full and was not taking no for an answer. Firefly was in the same boat. We stood on the deck. I got a visual of unconditional love and then loss coupled with a vision of me walking alone on a very rickety bridge over a lake of fire, a solo venture which looked anything but fun. I looked out and saw how far the bathrooms were and opted for the trees, safer, not as far and less challenging psychologically.

We went back to bed. A few hours later we had to pee again, but this time we opted for the bathroom, perhaps more levelheaded this time, I said, "We go together. Don't leave me no matter what." Firefly nodded and grabbed my hand.

As we walked, I could see residue from other dimensions – situations that didn't turn out as well, parallel realities, past lives, or a glimpse into other dimensions. We kept walking, hands clasped together. We made it. I stood outside the bathroom. "You're coming in with me, not just in the same bathroom, in the same stall." He replied, "I know," both of us recalling the cold shiver and the rise of hair on the back of our necks at Freezer Burn when I froze stock solid outside the porta-potties sensing something behind me – not someone.

As we washed our hands, my eyes drifted to the crystals surrounding the sinks that the bathroom crew had purposely left and I noted that the vibration level would be too high for any unwelcome visitors. Phew. I commented in gratitude and said, "Somebody else knows." Firefly nodded and we headed back to the cabin.

Inside he said, "Close your eyes and take my hand." My mind envisioned a minefield of psychological crap to wade through, but I didn't feel anything and just held onto the hand I trusted. We crawled back into bed, chilled from the freezing walk. Curled around one another, we were shown unequivocally and simultaneously that our primary partners were holding us back from growth. We were shown that life operates like a video game, but instead of levels it works with vibration and like the levels of a game, you can only access the stuff on your vibration.

The higher the vibration, the more awesome the stuff is that comprises your life.

Since Firefly and I had both quantum leaped, we had left our primary partners in the dust. What used to be a fading intermittent radio signal with our primaries was now just static. We were on totally different frequencies and they were no longer right for us to mix and integrate with. In dabbling with the energy of souls in lower vibration, such as sex, you end up lowering your vibration and stepping away from your divinity and into your human brain, which can't make sense of anything because logic tells you that security, the status quo, and comfort are far wiser choices, if not the best.

We were shown that by investing so much time, energy, and hope into having those souls come with us, we had compromised our own soul development. The time had come to choose if we were going to continue to prod, plead, and coerce these souls into coming with us, while simultaneously throwing our hands up in exasperation and banging our heads against the wall, or honor ourselves with self-love and take care of our souls' needs. We had to believe that we were worthy of what we wanted and stop sacrificing ourselves to help other souls, even the ones we were most closely connected to.

We were shown how consciously or unconsciously these souls had made a choice to be left behind for the time being and that it was all okay. It wasn't our fault. Our alignment, synchronicity, and connection were divinely guided and we had the ability to be more than twin souls with a fleeting physical connection peppered throughout our "real" lives, but to be transformed into a powerhouse couple if we were to choose "in." Twin flames are soul buddies, because the lessons that one twin is living out and working through is completely mirrored in the other. They have different characters and situations, but the exact same soul lesson. This creates a connection and a level of understanding between the two which is unmatched as we know what the other is going through because we are experiencing the exact same thing.

I turned to Firefly who had just downloaded the exact same information and said to him, "Well we asked for clarity. I don't think we could have had more confirmation if God came down on a cloud and told us in person our primary relationship contracts were over." He chuckled and agreed. We had collected enough coins along the way and successfully learned from our life adventures to achieve the next video game level. Immediately, our next task was delivered, to leave behind the patterns that stopped us from speaking our truths, the desire to keep the peace, or at least the perception of peace at all costs, which both of us had exhibited for all our lives. This new level was fraught with fire pits, mines, cliffs, and all manner of obstacles designed to prevent us from completing the level. The stakes had been upped.

In the days that followed, I saw those previous patterns which had held me back evaporate as I stepped into my knowing and my truth and now felt on firm footing instead of shaky ground. My path and my direction made sense to me and it was enough. I watched Firefly quantum leap again and step fully into his masculine self, a new role where for the first time in his life he articulated his own direction, took the helm, and started to direct his life where he wanted it instead of where others charted it through manipulation and guilt.

Now I understand the peace that passes all understanding and I survey my life in complete chaos. The tower had fully crumbled completely to the ground, dust still in the air, and all I could feel was free. The chains that bound me, guilt, obligation, "should be's," fear and doubt, logic and responsibility that were attached to my wrists by my own volition had now been released. I was the only person who could liberate me. Joy entered my being accompanied by the knowledge that the rainbow that I had been searching for after walking through rainstorm after rainstorm, soaked to the bone, I had now finally found.

# WAVES OF LOVE

## DMT

I was nervous. I invited a friend last minute to try DMT with me and she agreed. Another friend came over to guide us through the experience. He had us do about thirty minutes of breathwork before we smoked it. The breathwork alone had me so high. I felt amazing. He for sure knew what he was doing by preparing us.

My heart started to pound more and more as I watched him grab the pipe and prepare it. I had done LSD and mushrooms quite a bit before this but for some reason I was still scared. Scared to face my demons, but the total opposite happened.

I took my first hit and I didn't feel anything. It was a very awkward taste that I'd never experienced. I can't even describe how gross it was. I took my second hit after my friend and it hit me within ten seconds. I was instantly somewhere else. Somewhere I had never been before with any other psychedelics. I was completely out of my body and it felt amazing.

Immediately, everything around me turned into beautiful patterns and this amazing woman showed up who was also made of beautiful red patterns. Telepathically, she asked me if I was ready, and without words, I knew why she was asking. I said, "Yes" and then started to see her send me waves of love right into my heart center. I had never experienced such beauty on mushrooms or LSD.

As she was sending these waves she began to speak to me. She explained to me that all the love I felt I was missing in my life from my parents was never needed. That I already had that love inside of me. She said if I had that love provided then great, but if not then it was time for me to see the love that I am. As she was explaining this, she continued sending me waves of love. It was the most beautiful feeling I had ever felt in my life and I will never forget it.

She kept sending me waves and talking to me. She said these waves were going to release my fear and anger, but before I could say "no way" she already knew, so she started to show me a movie of all the times I didn't trust and how every time my needs were met. I was seeing a film about me right before my eyes. I started to put my hands on my heart and tell her thank you over and over again. I started to laugh in the middle of it all because I realized what a fool I had been to not trust and to be so full of fear. She showed me how fear was all a lie and although I had read it several times I needed her to show me.

My friend next to me started to scream "NO, NO, NO" over and over again. I knew she was facing something within her, something dark. My reaction was to place my hand on her knee, as all I could see was her energy, but not her body. The moment I placed my hand on her I said, "It's all going to be ok. It's all love." She screamed, "NO, ITS NOT! NO, NO, NO." I kept my hand on her lap to keep her calm and let her know I was there for her. But what happened next was exactly what I had come for.

As I had my hand on her knee, I began to see all the people

who had crossed my path in past lives whose knees I had touched during energy healings. It showed me that I had been doing this work for many past lives and that my mission was the same in this life as well. It was another mini-film of me watching myself healing others, but only quick flashes of it. I know my friend was meant to be there with me that night or else I wouldn't have had a knee to touch to show me the answers I was seeking.

As it was all ending, the woman who was guiding me told me that when fear came into my mind, she would be there to remind me to dismiss it and tell me that it wasn't real. That the pain wasn't real anymore. That I could finally let go.

I felt at ease. I sat there with my hands on my heart and she told me to breathe. I started taking in deep breaths and saw all these beautiful patterns going into my nostrils. With her mind, she explained that this prana, this breath, was full of creativity and it was important that I breathe in these patterns anytime I felt stuck. That it would help me to imagine these patterns as my creativity while inhaling them.

I slowly started to come back to this dimension. As I fully came back from my journey, I came back so grateful, so happy, and a changed woman. I had never felt so free and light. I felt healed in so many ways. I felt that most of my fear was gone. We sat around and shared our journeys, but I must say that the next few weeks were amazing. Everything had shifted for me. I was in bliss and so a few months later on Christmas night I went ahead and journeyed again.

# A NIGHT OF BEAUTY AND BLISS

## LSD

I was at Imagine Music and Arts festival on Orcas Island in Washington State. I had travelled there alone, as I couldn't find any friends who were willing to go and the festival sounded too good to pass up. The first night of the festival was great. Everyone was very kind and loving, so it wasn't difficult to make new friends. One of the friends that I had met and talked with for a few hours mentioned that he had LSD. I had some San Pedro cactus powder, and we agreed to make a trade. He gave me about one and half tabs and recommended that when I take it, I only take half to get a feel for it.

That night it rained heavily, and my tent was completely soaked. I almost left the festival as I had nowhere to sleep, until a generous friend offered to share her tent with me. I'm glad that she did, as the following night was the night where all of the magic happened.

I meditated for about thirty minutes to clear my mind, and then I took the LSD sometime around midday. I was sure to state my intention for the experience, which I believe is important to do before going on a psychedelic journey. My intention was for the LSD to help me become aware of my conditioning, my traumas, and my negative habits, so that I could heal them and be free of them. I also asked that the LSD show me the beauty of nature, and help me connect to nature and my own self in a deeper way. After stating my intention, I put the LSD in my mouth and let it dissolve under my tongue as I meditated for about twenty minutes, then swallowed the paper. I decided to take the whole tab and a half, as I wasn't sure if I'd do it again and I wanted the full experience.

After taking it, I decided to walk around. Orcas Island is beautiful and full of lush forests and a surprising amount of deer, as there are no predators on the island. The festival property was also right on the water, which allowed for even more beauty to please the senses.

I was in the art tent staring at various paintings when I met a very interesting and animated character who began talking to me about society and politics in a very humorous way. We talked for some time, and I remember noticing that the longer we talked, the more I laughed at what he had to say. The LSD was definitely starting to come on, but I hadn't done it before so I didn't know what to expect.

I began wandering around the open area where the music stage was and feeling the energy of the people around me very intensely. So much was going on all at once, and I could tell that the psychedelic experience was approaching. I began feeling a strong sense of anxiety, as I wasn't sure where to go, what to do, or who to talk to while the psychedelic experience approached.

I decided that the best thing to do was to go back to my friend's tent and meditate. Once I got to the tent, I immediately laid down. Not long after, my friend had come back into the tent, her hair soaking wet. I confessed that I was on LSD, and she told me about the water ceremony that she had just experienced and how healing it was for her. I could sense the healing she went through as her presence completely calmed down my anxiety.

She was curious about what I was experiencing, and we talked for quite some time. As I talked to her, the sunlight shining through the branches made a shadow on the tarp of her tent. The shadows were forming into a continually changing arrangement of beautiful geometric patterns.

As I talked to her, her face seemed to almost be melting. Every cell in our body is constantly dying and being reborn, and I felt that I could see this process happening as I stared at her face. She was a very kind and humble soul, intrigued by what I was seeing and not at all offended or weirded out by the fact that I was analyzing her face. Seeing the many facets of her face in such detail started to freak me out, until I looked into her eyes.

I saw that within her eyes was a being, and while the form that the being was in may change, the essence of the being itself remained eternal and pure. The more I focused on her eyes, the more peace I felt, and the less I was disturbed by the ever-changing world around me. Eventually, all I saw was her eye surrounded be a kaleidoscope of eyes, all looking at me. My ideas of "her" or "other" completely ceased and all I saw was my own eye looking back at itself. I felt strongly that it was the eye of God, and that I was the one divine Consciousness, staring at a mirror reflection of myself.

I have long felt that the essence within all of us is what we refer to as God, and I felt this more strongly then than I ever had before. We are all one formless Consciousness experiencing the diverse world of form. Within every form lies the formless and I was recognizing the formless Consciousness that is my truest self in the form of another human being. It is a wonderful thing to consider and think of, but a completely mind-blowing and beautiful thing to actually experience.

I cannot recall how long I was staring at her/my own eye, as time seemed to stop completely. I also can't remember exactly what we were talking about, but throughout the conversation I could only see this one eye surrounded by a kaleidoscope of other eyes. It was almost like having a conversation with God, a reflection of my truest self. This stunning experience was the inspiration for the cover art of my book *The Answer Is YOU*.

At a certain point in the conversation, she mentioned something about going to explore the festival again, and as I was still strongly hallucinating I began to feel anxious like I did earlier. She must have been able to sense the cause of my discomfort, as she stared directly at me and said, "You are the only one judging yourself." I heard her but didn't really pay attention as I was lost in my overthinking mind, until she repeated once more, "You are the only one judging yourself." This time her words resonated with me in the most profound way. I realized that I was afraid of judgment, not only at the festival, but throughout most of my life, in everything that I did.

I had been so worried about being judged by other people, when really it was just me judging myself. Throughout my life I had acted in certain ways, dressed in certain ways, spoke in certain ways, all just to get the approval of other people, when really all I needed was my own approval. When you accept yourself, you do not need anyone else to accept you. The opinions of others mean nothing when you are not dependent on their opinions for your own feelings of self-worth. As strange as it seems, when you accept yourself fully, others are more accepting of you too.

I completely let go of all judgment as I realized that it was all coming from me. All the fear, all the anxiety, all the stress – all of it was my own projection. Once I realized this I was able to surrender my self-judgment, and allowed love and freedom to flow into my being. I felt as though I had let go of a weight that I had been carrying all my life, and I had never felt more freedom, more happiness, and more peace than I had at that moment.

My friend decided to go out and explore the festival, and I decided to stay in the tent and meditate on what I had just realized to let it sink in. After some time, I could not help but notice the beautiful soundwaves coming from the music stage. I wanted to go out to enjoy the festival, but it was cold and somewhat rainy outside, and I wasn't sure what to wear, what to bring, etc.

I was hot inside the tent, but cold outside of it, and I was overthinking whether I needed to bring stuff with me or wear warm clothes and I realized that this thought process was the only thing holding me back from being where the music was, and so I thought, "Fuck it!" and I walked out of the tent barefoot, in a T-shirt and jeans.

I instantly felt cold, and then thought to myself, "what if I change my perception of what I consider to be cold?" Sure enough the cold disappeared. I changed my thoughts about my circumstances, and my circumstances changed. This was much more pronounced since I was under the influence of LSD, but we always have the ability to change our perspective of things. I am certain my body was still cold, but I no longer noticed it.

As I was walking from my tent, I gradually approached the sound of the amazing music coming from the stage. As I walked I felt free, alive, and confident. I was not worried about being myself, not fearing what others might think of me or how I looked. I was just content to be myself, and to allow myself to be myself.

I wandered directly into the crowd and started dancing. I have always been rather self-conscious about dancing, but this time I didn't care at all. It was so freeing to just dance barefoot on the grass to some great music.

Occasionally I would feel glimpses of self-consciousness, and would instantly recognize them as me judging myself. I would notice the judgment, smile to it, and release it. I also remember thinking that if I allowed myself to be myself, then I would set an example to others that they can also be themselves.

No one should have to hide who they are to fit in. Self-judgment is a prison that prevents you from being yourself, and when you accept yourself, you break free from this prison and a sense of joy and relief that you never thought possible becomes your very state of being. So much of our suffering comes from our judgment of ourselves – feelings of doubt, unworthiness, not feeling that one is enough. All of these are toxic thoughts that limit us from being free.

I had never danced so freely. I was using dance as a therapy, a way to notice when my sense of judgment would arise so I could smile to it and make peace with it. If my attention was focused on my own experience I was happy and free, but as soon as my attention went outward and was concerned with what others were doing or how others felt about me, then I would feel lost. I felt that by tuning into myself and focusing on my own experience, I was tapping into my power. I was allowing the Universe to express itself through me freely, as all of us are divine expressions of the whole of existence, and by trying to be like someone else, we prevent our unique light from shining on the world.

After the last artist played, the main facilitator of the festival got on stage and told everyone to head to the beach. We all walked to the beach, and what was awaiting down there was beyond magical.

There was a man named William Close playing what he called an "Earth harp." He was on a stage at one end of the cove, with strings going across the cove to the other side, and he was playing them like a harp. It was a beautiful thing to witness. As if the night couldn't get any better, a man came down to the beach and started singing in the most incredible voice. He sang a song or two and then began singing out to the water, as if he were calling something in.

A boat lit up in the water – a boat that was made up to look like a type of sea dragon. Then, on either side were two platforms, each with a girl dancing with fire. The boats began coming in closer to the shore as the man sang out to them. They were being pulled by people in kayaks which you could hardly see as they had no lights on their kayaks.

Once the sea dragon boat approached the shore, a woman began singing back to the man. He approached her and grabbed her hand to assist her out of the boat. He then sang in the most devotional way to her, bowing to her, making her appear as a queen. You could see how happy she was and it was contagious.

Then, a woman came to them with two rings, and the man sang as he put the ring on her finger – it wasn't until then that I realized I was witnessing the most incredible wedding ceremony. They said their "I do's" and sailed away together in the boat.

After witnessing this event together, the festival was extremely full of love and good energy. There were only about six hundred people there so it was a rather intimate festival, not like the ones with thousands of people. I spoke to an older woman for a while after the ceremony and after sharing the realization that I had of my self-judgment, she said something that really stuck with me: "We're all so worried what people are going to think of us, but most people are too focused on themselves to even notice. Just do what makes you happy." I felt a lot of joy as she was reaffirming what I had realized earlier that night.

I was beginning to feel my feet again and they were freezing, so I decided to go to a fireplace to warm up. Once around the fire, I joined in with a very musical group of people. There was a woman singing a lovely song, and her partner beside her playing the guitar.

The energy of love was so strong throughout the festival, and everyone just wanted to share their presence with one another. It felt so nice just to sit in a circle around a fire with people that were not lost in their thoughts, were not trying to be someone they were not, or judge you for who you were. Everyone was just being, and we were just sharing our time and presence together.

In this moment, I was overcome with a strong sense of love and presence. I didn't care to state my point of view or speak about my experience, I was much more interested in hearing what other people had to say, hearing their stories, seeing the beauty of who they were, and coming to meet our shared consciousness in its many unique forms.

I heard stories of people's art, what they loved, what they feared. I felt the pain that we all go through as human beings living in a violent and oppressive culture. I saw everyone else as myself in another circumstance. Our life experiences may vary, our bodies may be different, but the essence of life within us was one and the same.

After feeling this intense state of love and presence for quite some time, my body began to vibrate. I looked down at my hands and as I did, a woman next to me said, "ooh! Joe's vibrating!" I don't know how she noticed it, but she put her finger out to me and I smiled and put my finger to hers. We then all connected fingers in the circle in this way and I inhaled and exhaled love throughout the circle. A satisfying moan and giggle from a few people across the circle was enough to confirm that I actually was sending loving energy throughout the circle – I could feel the connection so strongly. It was such an oddly profound experience! The energy of love was so pure in this moment, and I had so much love for people I had never met before, but felt as though they were family.

I remained in this circle for most of the night, talking, playing music, sharing the good energy. It wasn't until about six in the morning that I went to bed. There was a lot more that happened throughout that night, but the events I shared here were the most significant.

Not only did I experience a night of deep healing, love, and freedom, but I took away many life lessons. I realized that any form of judgment, whether it was me judging another, or worrying what others thought of me, was really a reflection of my own self-judgment. Everything that causes a reaction within me becomes an opportunity to learn more about myself. I also learned that when we allow ourselves to be present with our experience, we see it for what it is, and we develop a sense of love and compassion for the objects of our experience, as they are not separate from who we are.

LSD played a major role in what I experienced that night, but a lot of it also had to do with the environment I was in, the people that I shared the experience with, and the insights and knowledge I had gained in the past that I was able to apply to my experience then. I am not sure how I would have handled the experience without some of the insights and experiences I have had prior to that experience. There were times when I felt the energy was really intense and without an understanding of psychedelic experiences, it could cause someone to have a pretty negative experience.

I do not recommend that one should take LSD. That is

totally up to the individual. If you do take it however, I would suggest making sure you are in a safe environment and have someone you know there to support you. I took a risk doing it at a festival with people I had never met before, and it happened to work out for me, but it could just have easily gone in a whole different direction.

Psychedelics are powerful, and they are not to be abused or taken without a pure intention. I believe they can be powerful teachers and healers, but that they are meant to help us tap into deeper levels of reality, and are not something to do purely for recreation or to do frequently, nor are they to be underestimated. With the right attitude of respect, the right mindset, and the right intention, they can be powerful teachers. But if abused, they can quickly humble you.

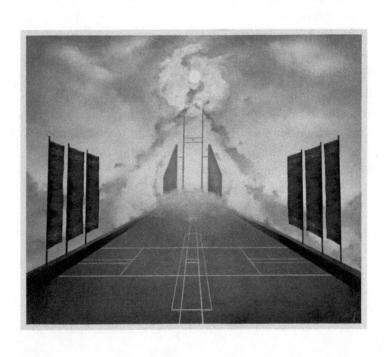

# INTO THE SOURCE OF DEATH ANXIETY

## Ayahuasca

I don't think I have ever really had a classic Ayahuasca vision after some fifty sessions. I haven't seen the Ayahuasca spirits, even though I asked them to show themselves to me if they were real. I haven't seen any DMT beings that I recognized as such. I have not visited any of the Ayahuasca or DMT worlds that psychonauts are known to marvel about. I can't say that I've ever had any real hallucinations on Ayahuasca, except for maybe a multi-colored energy flow out of my Crown Chakra, but that was real, I think, not some hallucination. My Ayahuasca visions on a good night are some color tones or patterns to some internal imagery that makes me remember early LSD trips, but nothing as dynamic as my best LSD trips. Most of my Ayahuasca visual experiences are just the things of ordinary internal imagery, something far less engaging than a good dream, some flashes of light or a couple of seconds of streaking colors and a really vivid image sometimes. Occasionally I get some sense of the "dot-like" graininess of internal images or the external world. But again, that is real, right?

So, if I haven't seen anything that looks like a DMT poster or a Pablo Amaringo or Andy Debernardi painting of an Ayahuasca vision, why do I still think that Ayahuasca is important? Because it has changed my life.

It began with my first ritual experience with Ayahuasca. This occurred in Missouri of all places, at the home of a friend who hosted Ron, a Peruvian trained American ayahuasquero. Our ceremony opened with a statement of each of our intentions for the session. I had pondered these intentions for at least a month beforehand, contemplating the need to address issues in various personal relationships as well as my own dependency issues and the need for changes in my life. The multitude of issues that presented themselves had precluded a decision, indeed all the way up to the beginning of the session. Still sorting through the possibilities as the other participants stated their intentions I received the inspiration to have no intentions, to turn the journey to the guidance of Ayahuasca. As it came to my turn to state my intentions I spoke in Spanish to the ayahuasquero and the brew, asking to be shown what I needed to know. I drank and sat back down to wait for the effects.

Ron was a skilled ayahuasquero who had been trained in the Icaros, the sacred songs of the Amazonian Ayahuasca traditions. The Icaro he sung first was something that he seldom sang, he later told me. "I sing whatever Icaros need to be sung, I don't choose them," he told me when I later asked him why he had sung that particular one.

The Icaro sounded to me like something involving banging metal pans together, beating metal pipes on galvanized aluminum garbage can lids, combined with a symphony of cymbals and gongs. As the sounds enveloped me a sense of nausea and dread infiltrated my consciousness. As I felt the clanging canopy of sounds penetrate to my core I came to a startling revelation that

I summed up as, "the world as we know it will end soon." I vomited. I was the last to drink and the first to purge. I vomited again.

As the Icaro continued I wondered, how did Ayahuasca know this? And the certainty that Ayahuasca had seen this happen before flowed through my consciousness. Waters rushing over the earth somehow seemed like the method, as vague dark images of Ayahuasca vines trailing up to the sky seemed to be revealed in receding waves. There were no other visions, no alarming words. It was the clanging of the Icaro that conveyed this certainty of the eventual destruction of the planet, the crashing down of the bastions of civilization. The world as we knew it was going to come to an end. Furthermore, I received premonitions about the death of my son and the end of my relationship with my wife.

The night had a few more insights about my future challenges, but the emotional content of this initial flash of realization was the most powerful and dominating. Somehow what I needed to deal with was this personal revelation of the necessity for preparing for the disappearance of all that we take for granted. The world as we know it was going to end in the near future.

I had not been an apocalyptic doomsayer. I had taken a course on the sociology of the future some twenty-five years earlier as an undergraduate, and had read the Report of Rome and other dire predictions about the future consequences of exponential growth on a finite planet, but I had not yet made any life decisions based on that knowledge.

In the spirit of full disclosure, I had been primed for thinking about a catastrophic event on my trip to Missouri, having begun to read Hank Wesselman's *Spirit Walker*, an account which he characterizes as a shamanic journey to his descendants in the future. In this book, he lays out a future world in which a natural cataclysm has erased modern civilization. He proposes that these will be the consequences which follow the Antarctic ice shelf breaking off and slipping into the sea, producing a worldwide tsunami that takes out the modern world.

I had stopped reading skeptically after a few chapters and picked up working on a paper for publication, so I had been primed for a view of possible destruction of the planet. I had also read the Wall Street Journal and USA Today on the flight out, absorbing the glowing reports of a healthy growth of the economy and the booming recovery from the 9/11 downturn. I had not taken Wesselman to heart at that time and was engaging my professional activities with optimism about the future. No sense of dread about the future was part of my conscious approach to the Ayahuasca session, but the experiences of the Icaro under the Ayahuasca's guidance had conveyed some wordless certainty to me. There was no shaking it. I was somehow deeply convinced of this inevitable reality and a sense that I needed to do something.

I might have been inclined to force myself towards something more rational, dismissing my visionary revelation as an aberration caused by my priming and drug experiences, but something else very interesting happened that night. An anthropologist who had done research on Ayahuasca wrote an e-mail to me during the night of the session, inviting me to come to Brazil to participate in an Ayahuasca conference. It seemed like an interesting coincidence when I read my e-mails two days later when I was back at home, but at that time it seemed like a coincidence rather than part of the message conveyed by the session. Still it was an interesting coincidence that could not be dismissed.

My family was less than enthusiastic about my visionary experience. As I had finished reading Wesselman's book Spirit Walker on the way back, I became more engrossed in his visions about the future. The breakup of the Antarctic ice was not a big news item, but the melting of the Arctic ice pack was getting some attention, part of the "global warming controversy" that was being challenged by many. The Antarctic wasn't on the radar – or so I thought. As I read the morning paper two days later, bathing in the skeptical concern of my wife who found my revelations a sign of a deteriorating mental condition, there it was: an article reported that a chunk of ice the size of the state of New Jersey had broken off the coast of the Antarctic and fallen into the sea. No big news, just a short piece on page three. It was news. Reading this piece of information in the context of my Ayahuasca experience and having an animated discussion with my wife Cindy and her sister about it fed my concerns, but what to do about my concerns remained vague.

My next experiences with Ayahuasca waited almost a year until I went to the Amazon. There, in a remote retreat center, I began to learn my way with Ayahuasca, a slow and often nauseating ordeal. Nausea and the fear of vomiting seemed to dominate my consciousness, but there was no vomiting, just tension in my lower abdomen and nausea. As I laid there in the lodge during the sessions I found myself listening to the surrounding jungle sounds and awaiting something spectacular. I was waiting for something that looked like a Pablo Amaringo or Alex Grey painting, peering into the darkness of my consciousness for some glimmer of radiant light, but the visions were not forthcoming.

Nonetheless, a significant experience did emerge in an early session. As I laid there in the darkness wondering when the wondrous visions would appear the person lying on the mat next to me began to moan. The groans became louder and more prolonged. I thought the facilitator would come to help but he was engaged with a number of other people at the moment. It reached a point at which something within me propelled me to act. I rolled over and approached the mattress of Andy who was withering in pain and asked him what was wrong. "There are darts in my stomach," he moaned. The Ayahuasca apparently activated the healer within me, as I intuitively began to twist my hand into his stomach to find and remove the darts which I flung towards the Amazon River. I worked for a few minutes finding several hard tight objects which seemed to dissolve as I worked them into my hand and pulled them out. As I proceeded, Andy fell quiet and the facilitator arrived to finish the healing. I felt an urge to go to the river to wash my hands in the cool water, removing whatever effects might have become attached to me.

The incident triggered awareness that I had sporadically experienced darts in myself, lodged in my back. Following that

266

session their sensations appeared, as a sharpened awareness of my body emerged. I told our leader about the sensations and he agreed to work on me during the following session. That night, I reminded him and he came over to work on me. Before he started, the sensations of the darts were strong, even painful. He intuitively went exactly to the points and pulled something out. As he did, the face of my ex-wife appeared in my awareness and the option to send the darts back to her emerged into my consciousness. I decided in an instant to instead send the darts to the cooling waters of the Amazon. The sensations that had plagued me for some years disappeared and did not return.

Intrigued I approached my next retreat with Ayahuasca with a sense of an explorer entering new territory. It was a research retreat in which I had the opportunity to participate in an EEG study that was performed outside of the sessions. The team was in novel territory in trying to acclimate to new equipment and to the situation of Ayahuasca. I volunteered to be the first subject, someone experienced with both Ayahuasca and being a participant in an electroencephalogram (EEG) study who could help them work out the bugs in the protocol and coordination as a team. I found the Ayahuasca surprisingly kind to me, with no nausea. The table where I had to lie virtually immobile with electrodes pasted to my scalp left me feeling a little cramped, almost claustrophobic. I focused on breathing and meditation in order to remain relaxed. It was also a back to back session for me and I was a little exhausted from the night before, enabling me to relax and drift into semi-consciousness.

The protocol had programmed periods of monitoring

rather than constant measurement and the opportunity to ask the equipment team to measure specific episodes we thought of special significance. During one of the non-measurement periods I experienced a flow of energy through my head. It seemed to surge out of my body along my spine and up to my Crown Chakra. As I lay there focusing on the experience, I perceived my own head as a swirl of energy that was shooting out of my Crown Chakra like a fountain. It was ecstatic. As I lay engrossed in the experience I remembered the EEG study. We were in a period of not doing measurement. I struggled for some time to come up to the level of consciousness where I could say something to them about turning on the EEG recorder. The effort to communicate and the experience were incompatible and it dissolved as I finally found the force to speak. I tried to return to it once they started the equipment but the moment was lost. And so was much of the rest of the retreat.

It seemed that session after session I laid in darkness, barely containing my nausea and enduring the knotted sensation in my lower abdomen. I set my intentions and gave myself over to Ayahuasca on alternating sessions, but was left disappointed. Ayahuasca was to leave me in darkness. It seemed that there was nothing for me to see.

A little more than a year later I was again in Amazonia at a retreat. It seemed that I picked up where I left off – nothing but nausea and discomfort in my lower abdomen session after session. My intentions had been to see the Ayahuasca beings and DMT worlds but my efforts were to no avail. I only saw darkness, a wandering mind, and more darkness. I was getting irritated with this. In sharing after sharing, the other participants went on and on about the incredible visions that they had. I had envy.

In the next session I got a little brash: "My intention is to have the Ayahuasca spirits reveal themselves to me if they are real," I declared. The session seemed little different than the previous ones – nausea, darkness, and a wandering mind. One thing stood out from that session that had an interesting confirmation the next day.

Throughout the night I remembered many disasters that I had narrowly escaped, like when a truck almost ran over me, and several situations when I was almost busted for marijuana. I remembered another time when I narrowly avoided being electrocuted, and an encounter where a friend got me out of a situation where someone was planning to kill me. It seemed that the whole night was just reliving one bad situation after another. Nothing fun, and no DMT beings so it seemed.

The next morning, I left the retreat center early and took a drive to a local beach. After a short stop there I decided to head to the city for some business. I was zipping through the parking lot to leave and was about to pass the attendant at the gate and continue to the street when I saw him give me a friendly wave. I took my foot off of the gas and braked for a second as I stuck my arm out of the window to return the greeting, wishing a "bom dia." As I returned my foot to the accelerator to continue, a pickup truck roared past me a high speed, just a meter or two in front of the car. It was so close and fast I didn't have a chance to even brake to try to stop. The driver continued, oblivious to the near collision. I let my car roll to a stop, my heart pounding. I felt like I had just avoided being T-boned on the driver's side of the car by virtue of having paused for a split second courtesy.

It took some time to process the incident, and some more to put it in context. It was during the sharing later that day that the connection came to me. "Where are the Ayahuasca beings?" I asked. "Show yourselves," I challenged. What I had been shown wasn't some fantastic otherworldly scenes but just my own life, and how narrowly I had avoided losing my life on several occasions, including that morning. I decided that if that is how the Ayahuasca beings worked then that was fine with me. I've sure needed protection along the way. Who knows how many other times the disasters that might have befallen me were somehow avoided by their guidance and intervention.

My Ayahuasca sessions seemed to remain the same. Mostly darkness with a few gleams of fluorescent light or vague images. A lot of wandering memories. "Return to the breathing and focus," I told myself. But only blackness remained. Often it was the cramping in my lower abdomen that was the predominant sensation. I wondered why I did this to myself.

A year later I was back in southern Brazil for another opportunity to learn from Ayahuasca. There were competing demands for my attention, as I attempted to launch a research project to assess the health consequences of participating in the Ayahuasca churches. Nights were spent in the Ayahuasca sessions, days in the university with colleagues developing the research project. I was surprised I had energy for both. At one point, I didn't. As I stood outside of one of the churches conversing with the leaders about the project, I felt my energy leaving my body and draining into the ground.

A few hours later I was back at the retreat center, just in time for the session. I had a sense of weakness. My previous intentions to see the pretty pictures had been to no avail. I had no clear sense of purpose. I sought an intention and found none, so again I asked Ayahuasca to show me what I need to see now. The session started like so many others, with nausea and stomach discomfort, and darkness. I focused on breathing and meditation, maintaining an open mind and trying to avoid distractions.

I kept finding myself enveloped with the idea of having an affair with a specific person with who I had never been romantically or sexually involved with. I tried to return to my focus and intention, fixating on my breath, but the idea of this sexual relation returned. No visions of the person, no pornographic pictures, no images of sex – just the idea of having a sexual relation with her. I would return to my focus and intention and in no time at all the idea would return. I tried to focus again on the meditation, my breath, and intention of what it is I need to know now. And the idea returned. Again and again.

Finally in exasperation I blurted out, "Why am I seeing this?" and the next thing I said was "Because Cindy [my wife] is not going to be around anymore." I sat up in shock. "Where did that come from?" I asked and the response was "Ayahuasca." I sat there still in total darkness, the candles by the stairway in the next room my only light. It was 2 a.m. local time and I was lost.

I think I spent another hour enveloped in this fearful possibility.

I went to my room to collect myself and decided to Skype my wife back in the U.S. to tell her what I had just received from the Ayahuasca. She felt cold. "I leave for a road trip to Las Vegas tomorrow," she reminded me. There was a trade show she had registered to attend. The silence was heavy and suffocating. "We must do a ritual to remove this," I told her, and a plan emerged as to what she must do before she left early the next morning. A ritual of cleansing and release to undo this prophetic path, to provide something that would give her protection.

My vision was unsettling for her to say the least; it seemed to have traumatized her. She called me from her hotel room in Las Vegas that night. Everything was ok, but she told me that on the way she had unintentionally taken an exit off of the freeway miles before her destination in the city. She stopped at the traffic signal at the bottom of the exit ramp, perplexed. She couldn't return to the freeway directly and instead had to turn and drive a mile or so down before she could make a U-turn that took her back to the freeway.

What had, a few minutes before, been open traffic flying along the freeway at 75 mph was now a virtual standstill. As she inched along with the traffic she discovered a harrowing scene. A car was turned over in the middle of the freeway, with others mangled together on the shoulder. No first responders were on site, and the police were not yet on the scene, much less ambulances. This catastrophe happened while she had inexplicably taken the wrong exit and wandered back to the freeway. Inexplicably? Or the Ayahuasca beings at work? There was a world of possibilities without the confirmation that science might demand, but when one walks the path with Ayahuasca, such possibilities seem to be heaven-sent miracles.

I still had days to go at the retreat. The emotions were strong: a sense of anxiety and relief. I wanted to be with Cindy. My wife and I had faced challenges from time to time but we both felt blessed with what most people found to be an enviable relationship, a harmonious compatibility in spite of our many differences. We felt like soulmates.

Suddenly it struck me. What if? What if Cindy was no longer with me? This would then all ring true – I can't imagine my life at peace without her and after twenty years together I still didn't want to have anyone else. I even cancelled her life insurance policy because I did not want there to be any sense of a reward if something were to happen to her. That energy seemed all wrong. A half million dollar payout wouldn't blunt the loss or pain and I didn't want that sense of a reward if something happened to her to cloud my real desires.

I realized then that a risk might still be present to her. Now six years later I hope that has passed, but I still wonder about this progressed reading and the Ayahuasca-inspired revelations that perhaps changed what could have been a catastrophically fatal day outside of Las Vegas. How could Ayahuasca function like that? Could it help us avoid our cosmically channeled destinies? Does Ayahuasca somehow operate within these deep cosmic patterns and at the same time give us the power to change them?

The day after the disturbing possibility was revealed to me, one of the retreat participants came to me and told me that she had received a vision that I would be able to heal her, particularly her heart. I rejected the idea for a moment, but then reached out and placed my hand on her chest. She cried uncontrollable tears of joy as some emotions were released. She had many troublesome relationships in her past and somehow this contact helped to release her from some of them. I decided to do something I seldom do – I loaned her a pair of healing crystals I had worked with for more than twenty years. They may have been some of the most widely traveled crystals in the world, accompanying me on many trips to Mexico, Europe and elsewhere. She used them for the remaining days of the retreat and returned them to me the day I left. Sitting at the airport I removed them from my pocket and sat them on my lap, but I forgot they were there when I stood up and they hit the floor, shattering into dozens of pieces. They had taken many similar blows before but this time some other force seemed to have possessed – and perhaps left them. The lady who had used them suffered a serious automobile accident some four months later, her car turning over on an icy road, but she fortunately survived with little injury. I thought about the overturned vehicle Cindy had seen on the Las Vegas highway and wondered about morphogenetic resonances.

My journey with Ayahuasca continued. It was over a year later that I was again in an Ayahuasca retreat. My health, with a recently discovered cancerous tumor and a significantly compromised liver, seemed to advise against Ayahuasca, but after a couple of days of liver protecting herbs and vitamins I felt that I was ready to participate. My vision came as a dreamlike memory, a few seconds time lapse. I saw my larynx, held in my hand. It then transformed into the skeleton of the back of a chicken, to which it bore some general similarity in shape. When we gathered to share the next day, I was a little perplexed and embarrassed. I often feel like the orphan child when it comes to sharing – so little to say. As we sat in the circle to share I picked up the pillow and sat it on my lap rather than sitting on it. As I stared down at it I saw something surprising – it was covered with embroidered chickens and roosters. I pondered this, looked for interpretations in dream books and books about power animals. It seemed to tell me that I should be a spokesperson, providing a warning by telling people what was happening in the world. Roosters are an early warning system.

Thus, I felt that I should share what Ayahuasca has led me to do. I have changed my life. I quit my job, retired, sold my house and cars and moved to where spirit has led me – the central highlands of Brazil where I am trying to develop a sustainable lifestyle. You can call me a prepper, a survivalist, and yes maybe a doomsayer. There are a lot of reasons to think that the world as we know it will undergo some cataclysmic catastrophe and that the future will be something quite different than a continuation or extrapolation of the past. There are many reasons to think we should strive for sustainability, an environmental adaptation that not only prepares us for uncertain futures but also gives us a more harmonious present. This is what Ayahuasca has led me to do.

I had skipped recounting the year before. I might have seemed like an anomaly, a little out of place in my Ayahuasca journey. But it was one encounter that perhaps shook me as profoundly as my original Ayahuasca ritual.

I had the opportunity to do something I had longed for – an encounter with DMT. During an Ayahuasca retreat I finally had the opportunity for the experience and embraced it with enthusiasm. I did, however, revert to my accustomed patterns of entheogen use, setting my intentions, and I returned to a somewhat worn theme: I want to know what the DMT powers can tell me to help me deal with my marijuana obsession. It was something I had attempted to address at several periods of my life. Once a shaman friend told me, "I see marijuana like a beautiful woman who holds you captive in a cage. You are entranced with her beauty and cannot find a way to leave her." Maybe I didn't want to leave, but I definitely found myself wanting to reduce the sense of being owned.

I had a good sitter. Zak said he had probably sat for a thousand people. He prepped me well. "Hold it as long as you can," he advised. As I inhaled as much as I could and held the vapors as they penetrated my body, I remembered his advice. Every time I was about to exhale he reminded me, "Hold it." As I finally let the breath ooze out of my lungs I slipped away into nothing.

About twenty minutes later I was back. As if I had never left. "Well what did you see?" Zak asked. "Nothing," I replied. "Nothing?" he asked. I heard my voice speak, "I have to confess something to my wife." "So that is what you saw?" Zak inquired. "I saw nothing," I insisted. "It was just these words coming out of my mouth when you asked."

We discussed this for a while. Twenty minutes of pure DMT was a void. "I've never seen that," Zak advised. But he admitted that he had heard of people who had a total absence of recall of anything following DMT experiences. "I should do it again," I decided. And with no ceremony we repeated the process.

Again, twenty minutes later I was back. "How was it this time?" he queried. There was nothing in my mind, but I heard my voice say "I did sorcery to break my son's leg. Why did you do that? It was the only way to get him out of Mexico and save his life." I sat there perplexed, because it was not me that had spoken. It was my voice but from where the words originated I had no idea. The episode had again been a void. But my son had been pursuing professional soccer in Mexico for several years and had his leg broken in an exhibition game try-out when he was finally with the team he wanted to play for – the Leones Negros of Guadalajara. It ended his career as a soccer player.

I thought about it for a few minutes. My alleged sorcery seemed plausible. In the weeks before he broke his leg I had a repetitive dream about trying to trick my son into something. In the dream it seemed that I was trying to accomplish something good for him, getting him to come into a room filled with golden light. But somehow I also felt like I was doing something bad. It had perplexed me. Maybe I had done sorcery unconsciously?

I suddenly asked out loud "Why am I confessing my sins?" "Because it is what you do before you die," was the answer that came out of my mouth." I was shocked.

After I digested the idea for a few minutes I decided to do another round of DMT. I declared my intentions: "I want to see the circumstances of my death and how to undo them."

This episode was more conscious. I seemed to "come up" to remember things and then descend back into the void. It seemed that with a change of plans, I had avoided some possible catastrophe. I needed to cancel my plans for Burning Man to avoid another, and finally I saw that an agent had been sent to kill me. It seemed that I knew with certainty that it was the "technological advisor" associated with the U.S. Embassy in Brasilia who had recently sought me out at a mushroom conference.

I came to consciousness with Zak attempting to calm me down. I was hooting in an ear-shattering roar. My wife sleeping some forty yards away was awakened, certain it was my voice. I must have awakened others. The following day I discussed this with several people. Tom, one of the retreat participants, had a chilling account. Literally.

"I had awoken during the night with a deep chill" Tom said. "I covered myself with two blankets but I could not get warm. I was shaking. I crawled into a fetal position shivering. I felt afraid. I realized that the fear was not mine. I experienced the fear as paranoia. I realized that I did not have anything to be afraid of or paranoid about. I put a bubble of protection around myself and went into a meditative state. When I returned from the meditative state I was no longer afraid and was no longer cold. I threw off both blankets and lay in bed trying to understand what had happened. I heard a voice tell me to leave the room. I did not want to get up, dress and go outside in what seemed like the middle of the night. The voice told me a second time to to leave the room. For a second time, I did not get up. The voice said you must leave the room now. I got up and left the room. As I was walking down the exterior stairs I could hear you hyperventilating in the room below mine and thought 'Michael is having a hard time.' I walked to an outside seating area and waited. I knew that you were engaged in some type of psychic struggle. After what seemed about twenty minutes the tension in my gut went away. I walked back to our house. I could not hear you. I went to bed."

We discussed this. "I believe that I was feeling the energy and tension that was coming from you or through you or to you," Tom said. "But I did not hear you until I had left my room." It seemed that his reaction had been to me, as he thought he had been awakened by my noise. But this was at 3 a.m. according to him and my session had ended at 11 p.m. It seemed that there was something unreal.

The rest of my sessions in the retreat were dominated with the concerns of how to prepare for avoiding my death. Tom was responsive to my concerns and in his next session he seemed to encounter the source of my fears.

"You're right," he told me. "I saw the guy. Pure evil. I looked him in the eye and told him to back off. I said 'If you do anything to Michael I will hunt you and your family down. And it won't be pretty. You'll be sorry you ever did anything.' Then I hit him with a bolt of power. He disappeared."

Tom was an ex-police captain with a steely confidence that gave me some sense of relief, but his confirmation of my fears wasn't exactly settling. I wafted between wanting to be temporarily delusional and accept that this acute psychotic episode would eventually pass versus trying to figure out how to confront this possibility of an assassin. I remained vigilant for weeks, wondering who might show up at the door. I bought guns, took a course in weapons use and got a concealed weapons permit.

As with many fears, this too subsided with time. Tom was also instrumental in that regard. We exchanged emails and a few months later he told me: "If someone wanted you dead you'd be dead by now."

And so, this episode remained as a distant reminder of how easily we can be led into our fears under these powerful substances. The notion that someone was sent to kill me seemed gone, until the day I finished writing about my Ayahuasca journey before the DMT experience. As fate would have it, I returned that very night to a session with Ayahuasca. In writing my account I had left the DMT experience out, consciously separating it from Ayahuasca. When I went to the session that night, my intention for the work was to address the emotional legacy of my father and the negative emotions that I still carried from the relationship.

The brew was good. I had fasted and the effects came on strongly. It seemed that after a few floating colors passed I was again engrossed in my nightmare – someone was coming to kill me. I saw a familiar but unknown face and ran through the thoughts that I had previously had about how to escape, confront, and accept my killer. Then another face appeared. My gardener! As unlikely as the scenario seems now, I was caught up and engrossed. I planned how I would confront him when he returned to work. I was so engrossed that even the request to translate from English to Portuguese for the session did not bring me out of the obsession. I translated virtually unconsciously, responding to the leader's English statements with a stream of good Portuguese, but remaining oblivious to people calling for me by name!

When my turn for healing came I shared my concerns, and the ayahuasquero informed me that there were two spirits embedded in me. As he removed them, one was screaming that it was going to kill me, but I remember none of this, being informed of it a few weeks later when he had reviewed a tape of the session.

In the meantime, I tried to remain calm and avoid dwelling on this obsession. But it was real to me and remained. I turned to my friend Khat for some help, either from her professional side as a psychologist or as a psychic. I got both.

"Michael, I believe it is your fear of death, not just physical death, but of total annihilation of the self, of the soul, that is pursuing you. Ayahuasca just pointed it out and personified it. I do not know how or why that fear originated in you, only that it is there. It haunts you and you have run from it: with pot, with intellectual affiliation, with changing locations. Still that fear pursues you, with cancer, with murderous neighbors, and with hungry ghosts that feed on fear."

Stan Grof talks extensively of this fear showing up dramatically in psychedelic states. He conceives of it from a transpersonal and/or perinatal perspective: "The transition from birth matrix III to birth matrix IV contributes to the spectrum of psychotic experiences sequences of psycho spiritual death and rebirth, apocalyptic visions of destructions and re-creation of the world and scenes of the Last Judgment. "Another source of paranoid states is the beginning phase of the second perinatal matrix… The source of danger cannot be identified and remains unknown. The individual then tends to project these feelings on some threatening situation in the external world- to secret plots or organizations or potential or actually dangerous human groups. The specific content of these frightening experiences can be drawn from corresponding areas of the collective unconscious."

Our experiences are often projections of our own unconscious fears and beliefs upon the material world, upon people and situations. For instance, a person experiencing a panic attack has a strong sense of impending doom, a doom that almost seems supernatural. These feelings are often attributed to specific places, ordinary places like highways and bridges, crowded theaters and restaurants or to simply being outside their own home.

For eons, there have been those that have felt with absolute certainty that the end of the world was imminent. This belief and its accompanying feeling state was so utterly convincing that they moved to caves or other continents, gave up all their worldly possessions, and left their friends and doubting families so as to save themselves and avoid annihilation. In extreme cases, they killed themselves and their loved ones in order to avoid what to them would be agonizing suffering and destruction. Yet the world and themselves, short of suicide, went on.

One cannot run from the fear of death, or for that matter any fear. To do so only tends to give the fear a greater strength and the opportunity to appear in new and previously unsuspected places. Fear must be confronted, the origins of fear identified, and the unseen made seen, while at the same time the power given over to fear reclaimed by the courage to face and deal with it no matter what the imagined cost.

In the shamanic tradition, it is often dealt with by surrendering, allowing oneself to embrace, be engulfed by, and consumed in the perceived dissolution-dismembered. In so doing, one can find oneself "re-membered" and reconstructed in a new way, the energy given to fear transformed. The experience of death is vivified and resolved in the experience of rebirth.

The notion of my fear of being killed representing a death and rebirth manifestation made some sense to me. The famed scholar of shamanism Mircea Eliade had pointed out that selection for the role of the shaman generally involved a period of illness, characterized as an attack by the spirits. This illness or a spirit attack was seen as leading to a personal death, often experienced as dismemberment or being devoured by animals. These entities may attack the initiate, devouring the body piece by piece. A recurrent motif is the removal of the eyes and their strategic placement for the observation of the total dismemberment and destruction of the body. The skeleton may be stripped of all flesh and cleaned, while flesh and organs are consumed by different mythological entities.

Following death, the body of the initiate is then remembered, or reconstructed, during which various animals may enter the body in a process that imbues the shaman with animal power and spirit allies. During this period, the spirits give the initiates new rules for life that heal the individual, and in the process make him or her a shaman, a "wounded healer."

This personal death reflects the fragmentation of the ego, which Dr. Roger N. Walsh, who wrote The Spirit of Shamanism, analyzes as a process of psychological transformation. The cross-culturally recurrent aspects of death, dismemberment, and rebirth represent deep archetypal processes in response to the inability of the psyche to maintain balance. The death-rebirth experiences reflect the death of one identity in development of another. As a consequence of the inability of the existing psychological structures to manage the stress, the organization of the psyche – identity, beliefs, habits, and conditioning – collapses. This results in a period of introversion, with the collapse of the internal structures experienced as dismemberment, an autosymbolic image of one's own breakdown.

Following the collapse of the psyche, experienced as dismemberment, a psychological reorganization follows, guided by an archetypal drive toward holism. Walsh suggests that the spontaneously occurring threatening images symbolize the shadow, aspects of the self and the psyche that are disowned and repressed because they are considered to be bad and evil. When these structures re-elevate into consciousness, they may be perceived as threatening external entities. The development of the shaman involves assimilation of these structures into a new more complete personality, leading to transcendence in a new level of identity. The universal experience of soul flight symbolizes this transformative experience.

Walsh notes that death-rebirth experiences frequently result in dramatic alleviation of psychosomatic, emotional, and interpersonal problems resistant to previous psychotherapy, with reorganization guided by archetypal drives toward wholeness. These psychological disturbances are often followed by increased mental health, a consequence of the growth experiences that they provoke.

These shamanic experiences of death and rebirth are not intrinsic signs of psychopathology but represent innate structures of the collective unconscious. These shamanic structures have been examined by Grof, based on his decades of supervising more than 20,000 shamanistic sessions with people from diverse cultures using holotropic breathwork and psychedelics. In addition to the biographical level of consciousness created in a person's experiences from infancy onward, there are two other major levels of consciousness – the perinatal and the transpersonal. The perinatal level reflects birth trauma experiences; while the transpersonal levels reflect dimensions of consciousness that extend beyond a person's body and ego. Both of these levels of consciousness are central to death and rebirth experiences. Shamanistic techniques for altering consciousness reveal these aspects of the deep structures of human consciousness and psyche, providing the organism with mechanisms "to free the bonds of various traumatic imprints and limitations, heal itself, and reach a more harmonious way of functioning."

Grof described these structures as organizing the psyche and the unconscious with themes fundamental to both positive and negative emotional experiences of life, particularly, anxiety, fury, pain, and suffocation. He analyzed perinatal phenomena as involving four distinct experiential phases or matrices as structures of the unconscious: (1) the amniotic universe; (2) cosmic engulfment; (3) the death-rebirth struggle; and (4) death and rebirth.

The death and rebirth experience is a culmination of the struggle of "'ego death,' an experience of total annihilation on all levels – physical, emotional, intellectual, and spiritual," according to Grof. He characterized this loss as the death of one's paranoid aspects, or one's false egos that view the world as dangerous and that feel the need to be in control to guard against danger. The sense of rebirth that follows this release from fear produces a sense of great energy, which may be interpreted as light, pure god, or unitive feeling of reunion with the true self.

The shaman's path embraced both death and rebirth; one must die in one aspect of self in order to be able to embrace a new development. Notably both of my experiences involving a fear of death or being killed occurred in sessions where my intentions were focused on change – overcoming my chemical dependency and my emotional baggage from my father. Truly something needs to die for a new self to emerge.

The idea that my fear of being killed reflected some manifestation of the shamanic path and the classic death and rebirth phenomena made some sense, but was not convincing. I had long recognized that my shamanic development path had stopped short of that classic experience. Furthermore, my intentions to address my addictive tendencies and my father's emotional legacy implied an engagement with a process of self-renewal and transformation characteristic of the death and rebirth process. My concerns were not from a death experience, just a fear of an actual death. I couldn't bring myself to accept this shamanic death and rebirth cycle as an explanation for my experiences, and it certainly didn't provide any relief from the lingering fear that someone might come kill me, as unlikely as it seemed to the rational mind.

Khat had told me one other thing that should have been an earlier clue. She reminded me of my long preoccupation with death and destruction, the feeling that death was stalking me and that Ayahuasca was giving me a warning. My major Ayahuasca episodes had involved the death of the world in cataclysmic destruction, my various close-calls with death, the feared death of my wife and son, the issues of sorcery, and then the two episodes of my own death premonitions (which occurred before and after a diagnosis of malignant cancer). Khat noted that in spite of previous work with MDMA, I had remained attached to darkness and a fear of death.

These kind of repeated experiences or reactions around an integrated theme were features of psychedelic experiences discovered by Grof. My fear of death theme represents what Grof called a system of condensed experience, or COEX, involving a specific constellation of memories and emotions. Grof proposed that our memories of physical experiences and the associated emotions are stored in these constellations.

287

Related emotions, thoughts, fantasies, and experiences collect together in a large number of clumps or COEX. Each COEX shares a common emotional theme or physical sensation. These themes follow basic emotions such as fear, terror, anger, humiliation, shame or loss, as well as positive emotions such as love, happiness, peace, bliss and even ecstasy.

Furthermore, he proposed that these COEX not only organize our individual unconscious but the entire human psyche, shaping our perceptions of self, others and the external world and leading us to behave in ways that fulfill those expectations. The COEX is the script that shapes perception and behavior in ways that recreate the same dynamics in the external world.

Grof noted that, "Of particular importance are systems involving life-threatening experiences or memories where our physical well-being was clearly at risk... In non-ordinary states [of consciousness] there is an automatic selection of the most relevant and emotionally charged materials from the person's unconscious... reveal[ing] aspects of the biographical realm that had previously eluded us." Tom, the ex-police captain, noted that these COEX systems are what Jungians (followers of the works of the famous psychoanalyst Carl Jung) call complexes. They have considerable integrity and stability, constituting the basic personality structure at a deep level of the mind. COEX systems link common experiences, sometimes beginning with the relevant birth experiences that have similar emotional and physical feelings. COEX systems also function as a basic disposition to the personality, linking emotions together in a strongly charged network. For instance, someone may overreact to a small annoyance, treating it as if it were a major threat because some feature of the situation, or the annoyance response itself activates a COEX. Any particular experience within one's personal history level will also activate its corresponding parts on the perinatal level, as well as across one's personal history.

Khat had elaborated on this dynamic, noting "that in everyday life our fears can create a filter; or rather our belief in the truth of our fears creates a filter, a lens, through which the world is perceived. As the fear grows so do the number of places, people and situations in which it is perceived and experienced. The more it is 'seen' the stronger the fear, the stronger the fear the more pervasive the situations in which it is encountered. In a paranoid delusional state, the projection created by fear is experienced as absolutely, incontrovertibly real. It seems an unshakeable truth. So if secret messages are being transmitted via a TV announcer, the phones are bugged, constant surveillance of immense proportion is being conducted, people are mere clones of themselves, that is, to that person, a fact based on how true it feels. The filter has created a total reality, dismissing anything not congruent with that belief."

"The shaman who told you that your fears attracted entities who fed on fear was correct," she said. "Whether we call them entities or lenses, the more we fear the more we attract fear to us. I do think that there are disincarnate beings in the middle world that are drawn by the scent of fear. Fear is their food and their familiar. There was even once a Star Trek episode that explored that theme. A disincarnate being that fed on fear infiltrated the ship and infected the crew. As they became more fearful and suspicious, the being grew more powerful. Someone eventually figured out what was going on, so the doctor injected everyone with a drug that induced a euphoric state. The entity had nowhere to go, nothing to eat. It was then trapped in a capsule and jettisoned into space."

"While the source of these fears may come from your early history, your prenatal or perinatal experiences, or your past lives, the answers to the resolution and peace you desire is within. You can't run from it because wherever you go, there you are and there it is as well. The unconscious within us is truly unconscious," she counseled. "We generally have no awareness of these buried perceptions and processes, yet they affect us greatly in our conscious lives in our perceptions and choices. Much as a black hole, dark matter, or dark energy affects our Universe, yet is unseen and unfelt except in how the Universe behaves responding to these forces, our unconscious affects us. Until that which is invisible, unconscious is made conscious in some way we have no way to observe or modify its contents."

Khat suggested, "You should go inside, go within with a skilled and trusted guide by your side who, with or without psychedelics or shamanism, can facilitate the work only you can do in confronting and dissolving that old buried fear."

A visit from Tom renewed this effort to engage with this persistent fear. As we prepared for an upcoming Ayahuasca session with Michael Bailot, we discussed how to formulate my intentions for best results. The notion that I should "get to the source of this issue" emerged as a good formulation. Tom proposed that we do a shamanic drumming session to prepare for the Ayahuasca session the following day. Tom and I set up the ceremony in our discussions during the day, deciding on a blended format of actual drumming and using a recording from Michael Harner's Foundation for Shamanic Studies CD. I stated my intentions for the journey as "I want to get to the source of my fear of being killed."

I evoked the powers of the four directions and the three-leveled shamanic universe with sage and began to drum. I was a bit out of practice and the actual journey proved a bit challenging to stay focused. The CD drumming helped. I saw corn, a pyramid, and the idea of sacrifice appeared. They had no apparent relationship to my question regarding the "source" of my death concerns, but dream interpretation suggested meanings of successful outcomes, pleasant changes, and reasons to rejoice.

When we discussed our experiences afterward, Tom was clear: "There is no one coming to kill you. There is no one that wants to kill you" he declared emphatically. "Death is not even on the horizon for you."

As we sat in the dark, the discussions that followed did however open up interesting avenues for personal exploration. "I remember a recurrent nightmare I had as a child," I told him. "It was about being chased by a naked man with a big screwdriver who was going to kill me. I think it was my father." Tom laughed, "That one is pretty apparent."

I told him about a memory that had emerged. When I was six years old, I was awakened during the night by the noise of my parents having sex. I went to their room to find out what was going on and was chased out and back to my room by my irate father. I ran back to my room screaming and huddled in my bed crying. My father never liked crying children. "I'll give you a good reason to cry" was often his warning before a spanking.

I am not entirely sure about all of what happened that night, but as I recounted this to Tom I had the vision or the notion that my father lost his patience with a sobbing boy. He came into my room yelling at me. "I'm going to kill you if you don't stop crying" resonated in my head.

I also recalled something else that afflicted me at that same period of life. It flooded back, the same room, the bed in the same place by the window, the same sense of terrified fear of my father. I had a prolonged episode of intestinal cramps that incapacitated me for weeks. They began as soon as I tried to get up in the morning, paralyzing me motionless for hours. Any movement to get out of bed left my lower abdomen with distended cramping muscles. While they subsided during the day, they returned in the evening when my father did. The doctor found nothing. I remember heated and incomprehensible discussions about this between my parents and my father angrily denouncing me for "faking it to get attention." His shouting terrified me, inducing further cramping and crying. I was never sure what the "it" was or how to fake it.

As we discussed this in relationship to my fear of being killed Tom smiled. "This all makes the best sense of everything," he said. "This is the most satisfactory explanation we have considered. You asked to get to the source and you got it."

Cindy agreed, relieved.

This interpretation presented itself as a very satisfying explanation of my death trauma. Discovery can begin to relieve the trauma, but it still needs treatment and resolution. As we made our final preparations for the evening session with the ayahuasquero Michael, Tom made some suggestions. "You have to go find and comfort that crying boy. He needs you. You need to console him." The idea of soul recovery occurred to me.

That night's session started smoothly. I felt a small dose was best for the healing approach. When my turn for the ritual healing came I started shuddering, partially from a sense of cold, but mostly some sense of energy jerking through my body. As Michael started working with the feather and chanting I started to relax.

Eventually my spirit guide Jimmy came through and started to work. He saw the roots of my issue in childhood trauma. "It is okay to cry," he told me. "It is good for your healing and release." A dissociated sadness overwhelmed me and tears flowed.

I became aware that I had suffered from susto or fright during that childhood episode. I asked, "Does Jimmy see the susto?" and Michael responded by additional pressure where his fingers pressed lightly into my solar plexus. "Right here," he said. He had told me years before that I needed to do some work on a blockage that I had in the solar plexus. I recalled it was a favorite point that my father had for poking me in anger about something.

Then I remembered Tom's advice. I found the little boy huddled along my legs and I picked him up to my chest, embracing and caressing him. Tears flowed as I told him, "You are okay now. You can cry." As I embraced him I told him that he was safe now and did not need to be afraid anymore. For a while we laid there, chest to chest, his head over my heart. Then the impulse came to move him over to the right side of my chest and he slipped inside me.

Lately I have experienced a sense of calm.

But I am still preparing for Teotwawki.

# 2001: LSD ODYSSEY

## LSD

It had been about four years since I last tripped. I had no idea I would once again come across the most profound chemical reaction. I had gotten back in touch with some old buddies of mine for a birthday party at the local bowling alley. It was great to see all of us together again, laughing, having fun, and finally old enough to buy some beers.

My best friend mentioned he had some "heavy-hitting LSD," and that it would be a great idea to go on a trip, like old times. It was getting late, around 9 p.m. I started to think about past times and how long it would last, but hey, when you're with old friends why not? He pulled out a small black tab, and said we could split it, since a quarter would be plenty. Unimpressed by the size and a bit relieved, I thought about how in the past small pieces were never strong anyway. I could handle this. I told myself, I probably won't get past the "euphoria phase," and I swallowed the tab with some beer.

We continued to share stories and finished a couple pitchers while everyone was bowling, completely forgetting about the tab. It must've been an hour or so before I realized I was tripping. I was slightly buzzed and needed to run to the bathroom. I stood up from the table and felt euphoric, completely in harmony with everything, still unaware of the LSD slowly working its way through me. I started walking toward the bathroom which wasn't too far, but the depth of my perception made it appear further than it was. After finishing my business, I was washing my hands, and a familiar feeling was starting to creep in like an old friend. I knew exactly what was next. I noticed the beads of sweat that started appear on the side of my head, and how light I started to feel, like my feet weren't exactly touching the floor, but ever so slightly floating. It was the LSD hitting harder than it ever had before.

I smiled, and got out of the bathroom and walked back to my best friend with a big grin, not really "knowing" how I got there. At this point, the both of us were beginning to trip. I already knew by the come-up that this was a whole different beast than I was used to.

Hours passed, and my memory of that time doesn't serve me well, but I made the drive back home safely, excited to hit the peak alone and try out new experiences. As I was trying to fit my house key into the lock, the LSD ran strong in my body. I couldn't figure out which side the key was facing since it was dark. I quickly remembered my phone had a flashlight. As I pulled it out and turned on the flashlight, I saw my key in all its glory. I was fascinated by it, for no reason. I put my key as close as I could to my eye and observed every detail, and started to laugh hysterically, as I realized it was the wrong key for this door. I got the right key out and quietly made my way into my room.

I instantly threw myself onto the bed, and marveled at the dark ceiling and the patterns that emerged, some blob-like, and others kaleidoscopic. My thoughts literally expanded, nowhere near capacity, but just kept on surging. The whole experience was a magnificent epiphany.

I left the window open to feel the breeze and natural sounds of the modern world unite and caress my body. Sound and vibration were observed rather closely, as they echoed through one ear and out to my fingertips. That was when I realized the truth. The Universe is one, period. Everything is connected.

In an instant, I decided to watch *2001: A Space Odyssey*. Only seeing it once before in 7th grade, I had thought it was the worst movie ever, but when the movie started I almost instinctively knew this movie was made for LSD trips. Every scene was actually synced for a trip, kind of like a "guidebook," but to sober minds it's just a really slow "sci-fi movie." I think Stanley Kubrick was trying to secretly wake up the masses with this film, without startling humanity, since a big percentage of human beings do not want to hear the truth about who we really are: ONE.

The intro of the film presents a blacked-out screen for about five minutes or so, at which point you hear a bunch of sounds that don't really have any rhythm or pattern to them. Just sounds echoing. For reference check out Tim Buckley's *Star Sailor*. It's really nothing but voices echoing in space. Then suddenly you hear the intro to *Also Sprach Zarathustra* with a shot of planet Earth covered in darkness. At this point you are totally present, in synch with the music and the slow rising presence of the sun. Then, as the song builds up even more the "Metro-Goldwyn-Mayer Presents" banner appears. Cymbals crash! HOLY SMOKES, I'm melting into the Universe, I'm watching the sun slowly revolve to the top of the Earth!

"A Stanley Kubrick Production" appeared. *Also Sprach Zarathustra* started to climax and I was feeling my mind blow away like that old famous Maxell blown-away-guy commercial from a simple magnificent intro to a masterpiece of a movie. I mean really, it was just Earth and the sun making their rounds like they have always been for the past 4.6 billion years or so, but I finally got it. Lying down holding my laptop up on my stomach, I watched the next scene unfold, "The dawn of man," observing the Africa savannah. Origins of life.

In this dark room, I had no identity. I didn't exist. The chemical had stripped me of my ego, until there was just a screen in front of me. As the film unfolded, I began to notice the nature of things. The apes wandered about and I saw them become territorial over land and water. At the same time as I was witnessing all of this I began to laugh. I began to laugh because as an observer from the outside I could see the bigger picture here. I understood the primitive problems of the apes, which in comparison weren't any different from the problems of the world today. This laugh was not just any laugh. It was vivacious and lively, a cannon blast from the soul.

Nearly on the verge of tears, I stopped. I asked myself, "Who is watching me, if I'm watching them!?" All of a sudden, in an instant, I had experienced infinity for lack of a better word. I saw myself over my laptop for what seemed like forever, similar to the effect of when you put two mirrors in front of each other. This was when I realized how we are One. We are all of time. Literally. Forever. Like the curves of the number eight.

I was slowly beginning to put one and one together...

just like the apes with the bones after the arrival of the monolith. The monolith was the screen.

This movie was the world's greatest joke, disguised as a film. It shook me to my core. We are all God experiencing ourselves subjectively. Don't believe me? It doesn't matter. Curious? Like Hunter S. Thompson said, "Buy the ticket, take the ride."

I also realized during this trip that love is the best. Love being our life, and self-reflection. We're blessed as people to feel love in its highest regard. It's just a matter of time until we see it as unity, to be as one. The reason for our evolution is to experience love and to live in harmony, defeating the chaos that surrounds us. That night it was immensely obvious to me that existence is all one process.

All my desires to be "somebody" had slowly dissolved. I saw slogans around my room from clothing, and different brands, and knew they were not me. These clothes, ideas, and catchphrases were false, but we have been conditioned to believe that they will make us become "someone," and that whatever we are doing is just fine. In reality, it's all in vain and it's all for the benefit of someone else. The ego has won when you lose sight of who you really are.

A moment later, I was gazing at my ceiling while lying in bed, surrendering myself to this inexplicable void – could it be death? Sure. I melted into the Universe, saw its core, a light of ecstasy, the origin of everything, love, you and me, these words on the screen all connected through an infinite love that passed through generations before us, a love that will continue to flow forever.

# DEPRESSION, ALCOHOLISM, AND AYAHUASCA

## Ayahuasca

I've decided to write my story. Everyone has a story. I didn't always believe in the necessity of everyone telling their story. I always thought that some of us should keep our business to ourselves. And, in some cases I still believe that sometimes we should. But who am I to say what should and shouldn't be shared? I'm just a huge fan of the "less is more" way of life. There is way too much clutter out there. And, with technology literally at our fingertips, there is more clutter now than ever.

It wasn't until most recently that I took a hard look into my stockpile of dreams and I decided to stop chasing them. I had an even better idea. I'll just start living my dreams by truly embodying the real meaning of living rather, than going through the motions. I'd been holding onto these old patterns of behavior and bad karma like a child holding her favorite teddy bear, afraid to let it go. It was time to break free of this prison cell once and for all.

Disease has become commonplace in our societal context and is sold to us every day, from commercials on TV, to advertisements on your subway commute, to the billboards on the highway. We are constantly bombarded with being sold a disease every single day of our lives. It is engrained in our psyche that it's "normal" to have a disease and that if we somehow don't have one, we should be looking for one. This is my story about my journey into my disease, my monster that almost cheated me of a chance to tell my story. I'm writing while holding gratitude for having a second chance at my life and being able to get a do over to share what I've learned in my lowest of lows and highest of highs. It's only now that I can finally sit still and focus to communicate without distraction or dis-ease to most effectively communicate what I've been trying to say for years.

Years ago, I was admitted into the hospital after attempting to take my life. I downed a handful of 800 Motrin with a bottle of Jack Daniels. That was my 3rd bottle of whiskey that week. I vaguely remember writing a note on a brown paper lunch bag explaining what I did. I had left it for my wife. The next thing I remember, I was in the back seat of my wife's CRV with our best friend being rushed to the hospital emergency room to drink a nasty charcoal liquid to absorb what I had consumed, then, I was admitted into the psych ward on account of admitting to the on-call doctor that I wanted to end my life. I spent a week in the hospital with other people suffering from similar issues and substance abuse. I had made the determination to get sober and face my diagnosis, which seemed like a life sentence: major chronic depression. The only relief in receiving that life sentence was now my monster had an actual name. I returned to my job after a week of group meetings, individual counseling and a week off resting up at home. I settled into my new prescriptions and proceeded with weekly therapy and regular med check-ups with my psychiatrist. After a month of being sober and feeling good, I decided to celebrate! Guess what I decided to celebrate with?? A drink! Imagine that?! I have all of this under control, I told myself. I can outsmart this monster of mine. I'll sure show her I can still have fun the same way I always have.

To my arrogant dismay, I was so dead wrong. Little did I know that I was headed for a bigger bottom than being in the hospital. I guess any rational person at this point would be saying, "Are you serious? Get your shit together. What are you thinking?" My monster had a whole other set of plans for me. Life has a very specific way of having you truly learn your lesson by recycling that karmic monster into an even bigger and angrier motherfucker than the last time. This would be one of the biggest universal ass-kickings I would receive in my life.

I tried going to Alcoholics Anonymous (AA) meetings. They were inspiring and daunting at first as it wasn't an easy thing for me to muster up the courage for, but I did it anyway. What did I really have to lose at this point? After a few meetings, I realized that this wasn't the path that I was looking for. I wasn't in judgment of it or any of the wonderful people I met there, I was just looking for something deeper, something that connected with my universal blueprint and spoke to me in a vocabulary I actually understood.

I tried a buffet of different anti-depressants. I went to therapy twice a week. Maybe these things could've worked if I was willing to let go of the old coping skills I had learned to use to mask my depression for all the years of my life. I decided to stay drunk and depressed and keep my monster happy and in control. I continued to go through the motions of going to therapy, taking medications and kept failing to turn my life around altogether due to my monster's twin. Guess what her name is? Yep, you guessed it. DENIAL! I was in severe denial of being diagnosed with major chronic depression. I thought that if I'd just get that promotion, make it big with my music or art, or just take a vacation that I'd be able to outsmart this monkey on my back. Wrong. Again. Technically, I suppose the week in the hospital could've been considered a vacation, however, that was not my idea of "fun in the sun."

We were unstoppable for quite a while and I was truly convinced that one of my monsters, denial, had that covered. I thought that I had everyone fooled. The only person the denial was doing a number on was me. She had me convinced that I had everyone else convinced. I began to lose control of the facade and fast. I was spiraling out of control. I was driving under the influence daily, endangering my life and others. I was mean, unhappy, repulsive, unmotivated. I was hungover all the time. I slept almost all day long. I was falling asleep in my car in the parking lot while going to grab some disgusting fast food to soak up the alcohol. My plan was falling apart. I was completely helpless and I couldn't see the possibility of breaking this vicious cycle. The truth was I wasn't trying very hard to overcome it because I had completely given my power away to something that was always taking from me. This disease kept taking from me because I was always will to give to it. I soon realized that I was too busy trying to die.

Once I made the final determination to get sober, that's when a tiny bit of light started to peek through in the darkness of my depression. I did one of the hardest things I've ever had to do in my life – face reality and the house I had built around it to hide from it. My darkest hours were ones I don't even remember. The person that is described in these dark hours, I don't even know. If I ever did meet this person, I'd probably kick the living shit out of her for hurting her loved ones so deeply as well as herself. The only thing I knew was that I didn't have the will to go on this way. It was either face the music and confront these demons head on or face the alternative: death. I began to paint again. I started meditating regularly. I began to research alternative therapies to try. I decided to give up drinking once and for all. With the help and support of my wife, our amazing friends and family, I found a community of support to back me in my wellness journey that had been waiting for me. I started out with Eye Movement Desensitization and Reprocessing (EMDR) therapy to unlock my subconscious that held the traumas, memories, and behaviors that I wanted the freedom from.

With EMDR helping me understand myself on a more intimate, deeper level, I wanted to truly heal the root cause of the depression and not allow the dependence on alcohol to run the show anymore. I was done beating myself up and reminding myself every day of all the things that I had done wrong. I wanted to look at these "wrongdoings" with true love, compassion, and understanding, without the judgment attached to them. I wasn't looking to live the rest of my life in the recovery world with constant references to the past, continuing to wallow in an unworthy state of mind. That's exactly what I was trying to get to the bottom of in the first place!

I decided to get my hands on as much research as I could about depression and dissect it piece by piece. I wanted to get to the deepest roots of it and face those fears and heal it once and for all. I realized that the self-medication and dependence on the alcohol was just a coping method and symptom of the real issue I was up against. I took to the internet and researched depression inside and out. I really sunk my teeth into my EMDR therapy taking it very seriously. I found getting to know myself through this therapy and research fascinating and wanted more. As my research and therapy deepened, I found myself always coming back to a plant in the plant kingdom called Ayahuasca in my readings and findings.

As a deeply spiritual person, this finding in my research was what I was directly asking the Universe for on both conscious and subconscious levels. It was the connection I was so desperately seeking my entire life. It was like following the same clues on the same treasure map and ending up in the same cave every day. I took this as a sign and decided to look further into the plant kingdom to get to know more about Ayahuasca.

I immersed myself in research about this plant and started to fall madly in love with her. It was even more daunting and inspiring than that first AA meeting. I asked myself why I kept coming back to this particular plant. This plant medicine has been used for centuries by the indigenous people of the Amazon to heal all sorts of issues including, anxiety, depression, PTSD, and addictions. I thought to myself that there has to be value in exploring this further if it can heal on this type of level. Then, I recalled a conversation I had with an old friend of mine about seven years prior about her experience with it in Peru. I remembered at the time she was telling me about her experience thinking "I don't know if I could ever do that," and "it takes a certain, special type of person to answer that calling," and "I don't know if I'm strong enough to go through that." Suddenly, it hit me like a ton of bricks! I was being called by this plant.

I put out my intention into the cosmos. I was crying and yelling out as loud as I could ask to make it possible to sit with Ayahuasca in ceremony. I didn't know what that meant or what it was going to look like. I had no idea what form this calling was going to take, but I trusted and handed over the heavy load to the Universe in hopes of her delivering in divine timing. It was two weeks to the day, I kid you not, and when I yelled out to answer the call, it all lined up. I had the details literally handed to me like it was sent by angelic couriers in exactly two weeks! I couldn't believe what was happening. In that moment, I realized that I was dealing with something way bigger than myself and the humility washed over me. I wept uncontrollably as my I felt my prayer to beat this huge monster that had been controlling my life was finally being answered.

I had two months to prepare myself for sitting with Mother Ayahuasca, as she is called in the Amazon. Having a date to look forward to kept me sober without any relapses. I weaned myself off of my anti-depressants, as they can interfere fatally with the plant medicine.

I was a hot mess of emotion, but in the storm of my ego unleashing all doubts and fears, I felt a sense of certainty and calm I'd never felt before. I knew that I was going to go through this and NOTHING was going to stop me. I was lucky enough to have two of my closest friends come along with me for the experience. That was just an added bonus as I was already determined to go, with or without the company.

My wife was doing her best to be supportive of my calling, but was also very concerned for my well-being and safety. I'm more of the risk-taker in the marriage as it's complimentary to my personality. She on the other hand, likes to play it safe and know what to expect. As one can imagine, it was very challenging to explain this to her as all I had to go on was what I had read and researched. It's very hard to explain something to someone that you haven't even experienced yet. I explained to her that this was my last resort. I was desperate to heal this and she needed to trust me.

As difficult as that was for her, she supported my decision as she wanted me to heal and get healthy again. Her fears were validating mine as well. She was scared that I'd be different when I got back. Maybe I wouldn't love her anymore. Maybe I would have an epiphany that my life with her was the wrong choice and I'd leave her. I just wanted to be free of the depression and dependency to ensure a better quality of life for myself, my marriage and my family.

The day of the ceremony arrived. I'd never been so excited to get there, get started, and get it over with. The two months leading up to this day had been like a prolonged twelve days of Christmas. I was dying to open up my beautifully wrapped presents under the tree. As my friends and I arrived to the ceremonial space, we were greeted by other participants sitting on their beds on the floor alongside their buckets facing the shaman's altar. My friends and I turned towards each other as I said, "What the hell did I get us into?" There was no turning back now. It was go time. We set up our beds and buckets at our assigned seats. The ceremony started promptly at 5 p.m.

The shaman sat down and welcomed the newcomers, as there had been a ceremony the evening prior. He briefly explained how he was going to dose and serve the Ayahuasca over the course of the ceremony. We were asked to state our intentions before our first serving of the medicine. Then, we began.

I sat in between my friends as we prepared to head up and take our doses. I'd never been so terrified. Little did I realize, this night was about to change the rest of my life forever. After everyone received their serving, we waited for the medicine to take effect. The shaman began chanting and singing Icaros. These are songs sung in Spanish to the spirits of plants to help them start taking effect.

About thirty to forty minutes into the ceremony, I could feel the presence of the Mother inside of every cell of my body. She had come to sit with me. I felt her gently coursing through my veins, my stomach, and my mind. I felt an ultimate surrender and laid down on my bed.

Soon, I felt the most intense wave of nausea hit me and began to purge into my bucket. It felt amazing to throw up and I continued to do so for about an hour. I felt all of my fears, insecurities, traumas, depression, doubts, anxieties, and addictions being flung out of my body mercilessly into the bottom my bucket. I felt freedom from it all! I looked at all of the demons in my bucket and said goodbye forever. After my hour of purging had come to end, that's when I began to sob uncontrollably for the next hour. I had been filled with an intense amount of gratitude, compassion, and love. I felt myself as a child being held in my mother's arms rocking me back and forth hearing the words, "It's okay. I'm with you and I'm not leaving your side. You take as much time as you need to cry. You need this."

The Mother was consoling me as I was being shown my life in chronological order, its genealogy, down to the roots of each generation. I was shown the pain and its origins in my family tree and kept saying "thank you" repeatedly. I felt like I was wrapped in a blanket of unconditional love, so safe, and so grateful. I clung to my blanket and pillow like they were my only possessions and felt immense gratitude for having them to hold. I felt myself going from repeatedly saying thank you to "I'm sorry." I felt all the pain inside of myself, my family, my past choices and the pain they caused others, and the pain that my family unknowingly carries. I felt one with it all. I was seeing it through compassionate, loving, and truthful eyes for the very first time in my life.

I finally understood the root cause of it all. I suddenly felt touched by a blissful feeling I had never experienced but always knew existed. I tuned back into the beautiful Icaros permeating the room, connecting me deeper to the Mother. I sat up and began to rock back and forth in delight. The sun was setting and the fire was radiating a glowing warmth throughout the room. I felt in love. I felt loved. I felt safe. I felt free. I felt so grateful. I felt forgiven. I felt whole again. For the next several hours of the ceremony, I was in conversation with the Mother. It was like a Q and A session, hearing her give me answers to questions I've been seeking out for what felt like an eternity. It was like I was being rewarded for all the hard work and preparation leading up to this moment.

I continued to unwrap my gifts one at a time, slowly savoring each second. I was so in each moment that it was almost impossible to think of anything else. She wouldn't allow for it. She had my commanded my undivided attention in such a seductive way, like a snake slithering rhythmically through the jungle that resides inside my body.

I felt her presence starting to fade slowly, not wanting to part with her yet. I could've stayed there with her forever. Before she slipped away for the evening, I heard her say to me, "We are just getting started. I'll be here when you are ready to come back. We have more to do." I felt like I was just made love to and couldn't wait for it to happen again. It was the most amazing and most profound experience of my life.

It was difficult to sleep that night as I was overloaded on processing all the new information I had just been gifted. I went outside and looked up at the stars in the night sky and cried. I felt overwhelmed with a sense of accomplishment, that I had just done something so important and life changing. My life was forever changed that night. I was looking up, understanding everything, but unsure how to use this new information. I knew

I had my work cut out for me in the life that was waiting for me to get back home.

The next three months ahead of me, post-ceremony, packed a brutal punch. It was the transition and integration that proved to be the toughest part of it all. The ceremony seemed like a walk in the park in hindsight. I found that the plant medicine was continuing its work with me in the real world. I had some hard times, profound shifts, hard conversations, and found myself really retreating inward to make sense of what I had done to my life. I turned it completely upside down, inside out, sideways and every which way. I felt alive again. I felt in love again with myself and my life. My consciousness was completely shifted. I was able to see all the same things with a new set of eyes, perspective, and a whole new vocabulary to describe them. My depression was nonexistent. I had developed a physical aversion to alcohol anytime I saw it, remembering the part of the ceremony where the Mother showed me why I do not need alcohol anymore. She explained that I used it as a coping method as well as self-medication for a very long time. I no longer needed that as I was entering a new frontier of my life that didn't have room for that.

The alcohol served its purpose teaching me what I needed to know. It was time to move on from that, otherwise it would continue to drag me down preventing me from realizing my life purpose and what I was called here to do. I understand that this may sound very simple. Like, "duh, who wouldn't be able to draw that conclusion on their own?" The message was very simple, yet I was shown a different perspective on how to feel about it. It was completely different from the logical perspective, a perspective all too familiar and hackneyed. She gave me an opportunity to be out of my head and connect with my heart-centered perspective which gave me the true power to release me from my disease and dependency.

It's been thirteen months since I had my last drink, as well as being off antidepressants, and I've lost over thirty pounds to top it all off. Talk about a snake shedding its old skin! My love affair with alcohol deep in the throes of depression seems like a lifetime ago. I've been given a true gift of living a life in transformation. I have absolutely no cravings for alcohol. My creativity is off the charts and I've been gifted with a profound and prolific time of creativity in my life. It's bubbling over with a new joy, meaning, and application. I've found a new love for my life, my art, my music, my wife, my family, and my friends. I'm in love for the first time as I found a new relationship in my life. This new relationship has removed the veil that was once shrouded with guilt, unworthiness, self-loathing, suffering, and death.

I have a new life filled with unconditional love, endless support, prolific creativity, deeper meaning and purpose in my relationships and a new-found self-love and a relentless self-worth. I am truly grateful for having been given another chance at my life. I'm beyond humbled to share my story with others in hopes that it may reach those who are in need of a new perspective on how to live again. You are not limited to your diagnosis. You can see it as a life sentence as I once did, or you can see it as a shiny new gift placed at the center of your heart, waiting to be opened.

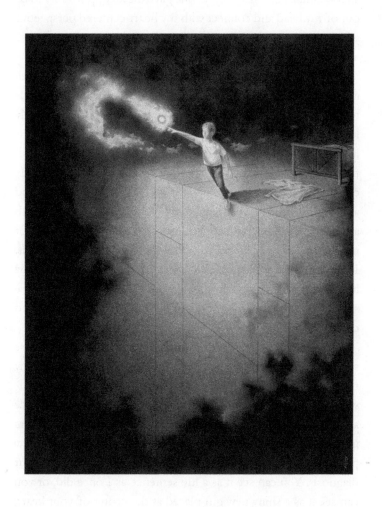

# COSMIC EXPLOSION

## Psilocybin

Psychedelics were not always a thing for me. Before experimenting with psychedelics, I never would have imagined what they really do to you. I had heard all the stories, but nothing like what I was about to experience.

I have always been really intrigued by the universe we live in. I would look around and notice different people seeming all content with existence, not really questioning it, but accepting it for what it is, plain and simple. This had been a painful difficulty for me throughout my life. I always wanted answers and for some reason I knew that I would never be as happy as the people around me until I knew the truth.

Somewhat of an outcast or an outsider, I never really fit in anywhere. Somehow I managed to get by. Marijuana was always a helping hand for me. I would smoke by myself or with friends and just enjoy the good vibes, and it helped me with anxiety mostly because when I was high, I wouldn't care about anything else. All my metaphysical speculation would fly out of the picture. By the time I was 18, I stumbled upon a little Psilocybin mushroom that would completely change my life forever. I wasn't really into the heavy stuff, but for some reason I knew this "drug" was special.

One night, one of my friends and I found ourselves with a half-ounce of mushrooms and a quarter of some high-grade weed. I decided to eat about 4 or 5 grams, not knowing what to expect, but I wanted to really experience the trip. We were just kicking back and listening to music. I started to feel a little happy and pretty soon the walls started to move like waves in the ocean. The music sounded a bit better and the lights were euphoric. It's as if I had stepped into some sort of electric dream where everything around me was alive. By this time both my friend and I could feel the mushrooms kicking in.

A couple of hours into my trip, I started having thoughts racing in my head, coming in and out at speeds I couldn't comprehend. It was as though the thoughts were visible, like rays of light. By this time I felt amazing, like I could do anything, and my friend seemed like he was having a good time as well. Then I took a wrong turn. I came across one thought that completely made things real for me. I thought about who I was and who created me and I couldn't find an answer. I felt this lingering sensation that something was ticking like a time bomb. I began to think about the history of our universe, the big bang theory, and really wrapped my head around the one question that no one could ever answer to me. What caused this big bang? I could literally feel all of time and all of space and everything in between. That time bomb was getting closer and closer to exploding. At some point the answer became clear but I did not want to admit it, until eventually I knew there was no other possible truth.

That's when it hit me. I knew I had somehow at some point created the Universe, but it wasn't just I. At this point I wasn't just Jason. No. I was every person that had ever lived, as one being. At the exact point where I became aware of myself, the explosion happened. I felt this huge wave of energy leave my body. It's like I was experiencing everything that had ever happened in our universe and it began to feel a bit painful. For some bizarre reason, the weight of the world was collapsing on me. Everything soon became my fault. All the evil that had corrupted this world and all the children crying were my fault. It was too much to handle and I knew this was my punishment. This was my hell.

The TV was on. We had been watching Courage the Cowardly Dog and there was a scene that kept replaying. I was stuck in a loop of what I would define as hell, but I couldn't accept it. It was like the more I fought the more it dissolved my being. I was in deep shit at this point with no way of going back. I knew I had hit rock bottom. I felt the pain of all the billions of years of existence and a tear came down the side of my face. Just one tear. That tear was like a sacrifice. This had to be done in order for the Universe to exist. I had to be here. In order for all the people to live I had to be in this loop.

As soon as I accepted my fate and I finally shut my mind, it spoke. Some stranger came from the other side spoke – the side that had seen the good that came from this plane. It wanted to show me the world I had created. I remember everything. The interaction itself was both frightening and relieving. It felt like some sort of dance. It was death and life simultaneously, dissolving my 3rd dimensional perception. The only thing to do was stop and listen. It was as if I had died and was reborn.

This stranger has always been revealing itself, I just happened to be looking right past it. I cannot describe this stranger or begin to know exactly who this stranger was, but I now look back at it as some guardian angel letting me know it was all okay and gave me a reason for why the journey has been worth the struggle. It was like dropping of veil, the unmasking of a hideous beast. I was the beast who had been unaware of its own darkness. It was euphoric.

This stranger had a terrible darkness to it as well, although it did free me from this prison where I had found myself being the guest of honor. This stranger knew what I was thinking and it knew the enormous amount of fear I had just coming into contact with it. This stranger was me, but it was also you. It's what lies behind the illusion that we are all separate. Everyone you look at is this stranger. You might see different faces but if you look closely it's all the same being looking back at you. Although the vessel might be completely unaware of this stranger, they are carrying out its plan. Their plan.

This stranger knows us all too well and will reveal itself to each of us in its own way, but all at the same. See this stranger is a being like any other. In fact, it is being itself. This stranger is what most would call God, but God is infinitely underestimated. We humans must have an explanation for everything, but this one cannot be explained. I understand this sounds a bit frustrating, but not as frustrating as looking for yourself. That's a double entendre not many will understand. It may seem like a curse, but it is a blessing in disguise. This stranger is as conscious as you or me and for various reasons that cannot be named, for it is without form or meaning, beyond time, beyond creation.

This being singlehandedly designed everything in our known and unknown universe. It designed itself. This stranger isn't such a stranger since it has been here all along, waiting patiently. It is a force which cannot be moved or persuaded or even understood.

In order to ensure every man finds their own way, this being had to sacrifice it all. Everything had to be this way. For it saw us before we existed and we had to exist. This is what they refer to as "God has a plan." Without us, it would not exist. Without your eyes, there would be nothing to see. If you could not feel, there would be nothing to touch. You are but a vessel for this being. I'm not even too sure that you exist.

This being is and always will be one step ahead. Actually, it is an infinite number of steps ahead and that increases with each passing moment. It has a sinister yet loving presence. As I became aware of this stranger, I was already too far gone. This being showed me a fraction of what it had seen. It explained why my pain and suffering is but an insult to it.

Just when I thought it couldn't get any worse. My soul was about to endure something I would never wish on another. In a way, this being did me a favor. See it was my opinions and all my questions which led me to this place. What I imagined was hell was only but a grid, a net which held me together no matter what. Once my perception had been cleansed, I had no more expectations of what was next and no more fear. It felt like I was being walked into heaven, into a world I had not been ready to see, until now. What I would describe as heaven. But it was here on Earth.

The sun was coming up and my friend was sleeping like a

baby. I went outside to enjoy the garden and smoke a blunt by myself. It felt like such a privilege to enjoy its luxury.

Since then everything has been great. The frequency has guided me and I have been extremely grateful. My life has been nothing but positive and all the negativity has slowly faded away. I eat better, feel more in tune, and I absorb and observe everything I come across. I have seen the light. I feel more alive by the day and I'm at a point in my life where I don't need anything. I am immortal.

I believe that for the months following my experience, I went through a kundalini awakening. At first, I was scared by how painful it was, but not to worry, the pain was worth it. I am no longer this lifeless corpse, but a warrior of light. Once a three-dimensional being, now turned into this eager child ready to see the world. All that's left for me in this life is to serve my fellow brothers and sisters. Misguided by many and lied to infinitely, I shall take matters into my own hands. Wait until they get a load of me.

# MY REBIRTH

## DMT

When I took the first hit, I closed my eyes. As soon as I blew out the smoke, I instantly felt dizzy and had difficulty breathing. I held a pillow in my arms as if my life depended on it. I clung to it and squeezed it hard and was short of breath for the first few minutes.

Finally, I began to relax and saw different visions, similar to those found in mandalas and mosaics. There were plenty of patterns and shapes that fit together, moving in every direction, making whirlwinds. I heard a sparkle, like when you hear the sound of a starry sky in an animated program or a bit like binaural beat. It was as if I could hear all the vibrations inside my body and everything around me. From an angle, I saw short flashes of images that were circulating, but when I tried to look at them, the images would disappear and repeat. I felt an intense sense of wellbeing and had the impression of seeing 360-degrees inside my head, inside my own consciousness.

The more time passed, the more I felt as though I were moving forward in space. I felt like I was traveling in my own head and I was going through different dimensions! It was really intense and it lasted about twenty minutes. I was in a room where no one spoke, but I heard so much more than usual. It seemed as though my hearing was fifteen times more developed.

When the effect began to dissipate, the visions and sounds

gradually disappeared. When I came back, I was speechless. I just couldn't believe it! Everything I saw was so beautiful, yet inexplicable. I felt like I had realized so many things, and now knew a truth that I could not explain to my friends. It helped me realize that there is so much more for me to learn in this life. I felt a great connection with nature, with space, and with dimensions whose existence I did not know. I questioned everything that we're taught in society.

It was a big feeling of wellbeing, but a big shock at the same time. The next day, all the sounds I had known were no longer the same. When I flushed the toilet, the noise was different than the sound of a toilet that I had always known. I had the impression of hearing the vibrations of everything that surrounded me – the trees, the wind, even the sounds in my apartment.

The day after this experience, I had a few days of mini depression. It was the first time I felt this immense void. I only thought about my experience and I only wanted to sleep. I had no interest in what I loved. In fact, I didn't like anything anymore and it really disturbed me, so I got a little down. After this little down everything changed. In fact, it was at this moment that I really learned to know myself and have interests that motivated me. It was at this moment that I found myself. It was like I was a new person. I became a more spiritual person, and so I impatiently waited for the day when I was going to try DMT again.

After a year went by, I finally had the chance to smoke DMT again. It was the day before my birthday and I was so happy that my friend finally had it. It was late and I waited until 11:55 p.m.

to smoke the DMT, because I wanted to come back to reality on my birthday. I couldn't think of a better way to celebrate.

I was both stressed and nervous at the same time. When my friend prepared my hit, he dropped a little more than the expected dose, but I took it anyway. I took a hit and held onto my pillow, but this time it was much different.

As soon as I blew out the smoke, I closed my eyes. I felt propelled much faster than the first time and in a different world than the one I had discovered a year before. This time, I didn't go through the dimensions one at a time with the chance to admire each moment. This time, I had the impression that I teleported directly into a dimension that I did not want to see and that I did not expect to discover. I was scared.

All of a sudden, I felt that time had stopped altogether. I was stuck in my head and I had the impression of reliving the same moment without stopping, like a video that repeats on loop. I heard the same sound of vibration repeating itself, as if I could hear my heartbeat. I had lost all memory of who I was and who my family and friends were. It was as if I were a baby again, born without memory, and without a past. I had lost my memories of my life. I felt that I was nothing and that only my consciousness existed. I thought I was going to be stuck here for the rest of my life.

I heard my own thoughts resonate inside of my head as if someone were telling me them out loud. I was unable to speak, make a sound, or even move. I was lost in my conscience and alone with my soul until the effects of the DMT began to dissipate.

I had no idea how long it actually took for me to come back to myself and take possession of my own body and voice, but when I was able to speak I said, "I am not okay!" I managed to open my eyes, because I wanted to get out of my head and that was the moment that I found the eternal. When I opened my eyes, it was all white and I could see nothing around me. I couldn't see what was around me in this reality, in my own living room. I had not found my vision yet, I was still in my head, in my subconscious, but this time my eyes were wide open. I couldn't see anything, so I asked for help from my boyfriend and my friend. I had a huge need to be reassured and heard them tell me that everything would be fine.

I started to find my vision when my boyfriend reassured me. It was so beautiful! On a white background, I saw colorful forms and patterns. At the same time, I remembered that I had a dog and I needed to see and touch it. When he came to see me, he was made of rainbow colors with lots of patterns. I saw this full visual effect everywhere in my apartment. My boyfriend and friend's faces sparkled like crystals shining in the sun. It was really beautiful.

I began to cry and laugh at the same time. I had never been so grateful to live. I was so emotional and happy to be alive. After this feeling of immense emptiness, I found myself lucky to be there in the present moment, as if I had relived my own birth.

# MASTER PLANT DIETA

## Ayahuasca

In traditional Amazonian shamanism, the master plant dieta (commonly known as 'La Dieta') is a process in which an apprentice shaman enters strict isolation in the jungle, adheres to a very limited diet, and ingests and cultivates a relationship with a particular plant in order to learn the teachings and healing modalities that the essence of this plant has to offer.

Restrictions differ depending on lineage, tradition and beliefs, however similarities exist. Generally the diet is bland, with no salt, sugar, spices, oils, dairy, red meats, fermented foods, or alcohol. There is limited contact and communication with others, hence the strict seclusion and isolation in the jungle. Entertainment such as music and reading are prohibited. No soaps, deodorants, toothpaste, or other artificial substances are permitted, and abstinence from all sexual activity is a necessity.

Traditional post-dieta protocols follow the same guidelines, anywhere from three to thirty days (perhaps even more) after the conclusion of working with the plants. Essentially, all of this is undertaken to keep the body, mind and spirit as clean, clear, pure, and sensitive as possible, so that one can notice the subtleties of the plant wisdom coming through.

I spent nine days adhering to a similar structure, working with both Ayahuasca and my master plant, Chiric Sanango, listening to and learning what the plants had to teach me. It wasn't without struggle. The process involved strong resistance on my behalf, largely due to fear and trust issues surrounding worsening health issues, and the cessation of contact between loved ones.

I underestimated how challenging this would be, but by my fourth and final Ayahuasca ceremony, I was gifted with remarkable physical healing, and many insightful teachings and wisdom.

The initial ceremony was mainly about cleansing and clearing space, so that my master plant, Chiric Sanango, could begin to enter and intertwine with my system over the subsequent few days. At 7 p.m. every night, we had a half hour meditation, followed by an Ayahuasca ceremony at 8 p.m. every other day.

A lot of bodily sensations were present: tingling and buzzing sensations throughout my body and head, especially my lips. At times, the pressure in my head was so dense that it felt like it was on the verge of implosion.

Eclectic visuals consisting of rotating green and yellow fractal patterns entered my existence, while humanoid entities flittered in and out with their ephemeral nature, seemingly void of any meaning or teachings.

As the medicine intensified, the focus of this experience was brought down to my lungs. This was no surprise. In my past five ceremonies in Australia, my awareness had consistently been placed on my lung health. Having suffered from asthma since my childhood, and having other respiratory issues for a few years linked to an unknown illness, the medicine was continuously bringing this to my attention. It was clearly an ailment that was holding me back and that needed to be resolved.

In between a few mild purges, I went into coughing fits, trying to bring up mucous from my respiratory system, hoping to clear the unpleasant feeling in my chest. Amongst all of this, an insight regarding clarity came to me. I kept asking for more clarity in my life, in terms of meaning, purpose, and direction. It seemed that this clarity was not necessarily going to be about illuminating or finding hidden gems in my subconscious mind, but more so about clearing away the fog and unnecessary clutter, so that what I already know and have in my life can shine more brightly.

At 8 a.m. every morning, my shamans came to me with the shredded root of Chiric Sanango, infused with water in a large mug. The texture and consistency was akin to thick sawdust, which was as one might imagine, uncomfortable to swallow down.

According to my shaman's perspective, this plant would stay in my system for six months, and if I completed La Dieta satisfactorily, it would become a plant ally in a psychological and spiritual sense for the rest of my life.

He told me this could be a powerful life-reset; a great first plant to diet with in alignment with the warrior's path. It would be a medicine and teacher to bring me more into integrity, to aid with direction and clarity, to allow me to continue cultivating the strong and courageous, yet loving and gentle warrior within, and unite me more with spirit.

According to what I'd read from Steve Beyer, "The effect of ingesting Chiric Sanango can be dramatic – a tingling and vibrating sensation in the extremities, moving inward toward the head with ever-increasing intensity; periodic waves of cold; tremors, electric vibrations penetrating the chest and back, stomach cramps, nausea, dizziness, vertigo, loss of coordination."

I was anxious and curious as to what I was about to experience as I proceeded to lay down in bed, becoming as still as possible, observing any noticeable changes in perception.

After about an hour, and for the following couple of hours, I experienced many bodily sensations, including numbing of the lips, tingling in the head and face, a coldness spreading throughout my extremities, and regular disturbances in my digestive tract, which led to a few bouts of diarrhea. The peak intensity faded after three hours, and I felt extremely lucid for the remainder of the day, with my equilibrium slightly off and my vision a little distorted.

By the afternoon, a mere two days in, I'd realized my incessant need to constantly be "doing," to distract myself from the onset of potential boredom. I had never considered it to be detrimental in daily life, however, I'm beginning to see where I seek out meaningless entertainment and distractions to prevent myself from simply "being."

I was glad to pick up on this – to try and break these habits so that they wouldn't transition into procrastination, in regards to the things I really should be spending my time and energy on.

Moments of sadness and loneliness were setting in and I released a lot of tension through crying, which alleviated some of the emotions I was feeling. This was stemming merely from the thought of not being able to communicate with loved ones, from projecting these thoughts into the future and reminiscing on the past.

One of the things I wanted to work on was to deepen my presence in everyday life, and this was certainly an ideal/ challenging situation to practice that.

The next morning, Chiric Sanango had no resemblance of sawdust, but more so a mildly sweet water that was easy to get down. For the first couple of hours, I was awake, yet in a dreamlike state at the same time. My lips became numb, but I was nowhere near as lucid as the day before.

During and after the peak of Chiric Sanango's effects, my breathing capacity seemed to moderately improve, but correlation doesn't equate to causation. Perhaps moving around in the sun during the day played a large role in how my health felt.

Overall though, my breathing appeared to be worsening. Even with an Ayahuasca ceremony that night, I took a small risk and used my asthma puffer slightly, several times. It is important to note that taking asthma medications and other pharmaceuticals could have severe and dangerous biochemical interactions with the MAO inhibiting qualities of Ayahuasca, and is NOT advised. With a heavy feeling still sinking into my chest, I thought it could be a respiratory infection of some sort coming on.

Reflecting back upon my previous medicine ceremonies, I was a little confused and suspicious. I hadn't quite figured out if the medicine was helping by bringing up stagnant phlegm and reducing inflammation in my chest, or, if drinking Ayahuasca was causing my body to become more run down – causing it to produce more phlegm and inflammation. My trust issues around my body and the medicine's capabilities could be a self-fulfilling prophecy into worsening health.

At the next ceremony, I only drank a very small cup, no more than a shot glass. I didn't want to drink. My health was on my mind. After the Icaros began, I left the temple space and proceeded to try and hack up anything in my lungs. It's absolutely horrible being in an altered state feeling like you can't breathe properly, especially when breath plays such a huge part in the experience.

During intense moments, to not be able to come back to the stillness and comfort of consistent and healthy breathing is extremely distracting and makes for an incredibly uncomfortable time.

The visual experience was mild, with an emphasis on consistent, heavy buzzing sensations in my head. I hadn't yet connected with Chiric Sanango in a visionary perception. I did have the sense that the plants could help with my ailments though.

Trust, trust, trust. I needed to trust. But that was the dilemma. It was challenging to trust and surrender completely when I felt like I was taking such a massive risk in terms of being in an altered state with poor respiratory function.

I could notice more resistance and fear settling in...

Consistency: sawdust again. With my labored breathing, congested sinuses, and constant sneezing, I was praying that the plants could help heal me.

Amongst the body chills and tingling in my extremities, this was the first time I could feel a strong vibrational pulse coursing through my body, a constant buzz. When I held my hand up to my face to observe the shaking, I couldn't notice much, but inside it felt like my central nervous system was hooked up to a super-charged battery.

I was feeling deeply humbled by how difficult all of this was. In all honesty, the thought of ending this prematurely found its way into my mind several times, yet I was beginning to see how undertaking and completing this journey was a real testament to the resilience of my character and spirit.

Although I'd been broken down several times and let my emotions get the best of me, a new foundation of strength, love, kindness and softness was beginning to form. I was pulling out the weeds, and planting new seeds to nurture and grow.

It was the final morning of ingesting Chiric Sanango. Apparently it's too taxing on the body to continue on with high doses, so we were given a little less than half the dosage of the day before, tapering us off smoothly (although it didn't make it any easier swallowing the sawdust down again). Similarly, there was coldness in my fingers and toes, and the vibrational pulse was present, although not as strong as the day before. I was quite spaced out and lucid, carrying a minor headache.

Chiric Sanango is also an aphrodisiac, which would explain some of the dreams I'd been having. It's challenging to alleviate and steer away from these feelings as soon as they arise, as sexual thoughts are prohibited in a purely traditional shamanistic context. In fact, it's said that an apprentice shaman's maestro is able to look into their apprentice's eyes to see if they've given in to the temptations of sexual thoughts, which would result in the termination of the apprenticeship. They would never be permitted to become a pure master shaman with only positive intentions for healing.

Going further down the rabbit hole, it's said that these failed apprentices would become known within their community to have failed their training, and would perhaps harbor resentment and envy toward others, which would generally lead to the practice of brujeria, black magic and witchcraft, which is the practice of negative intentions within the shamanistic context.

The way I saw it, sexual energy of any kind could be very overpowering and strong, and didn't allow for the subtleties of the plant energy to be observed as acutely. Sexual thoughts or behaviors can also give way to desire; not a feeling I wanted to indulge in when trying to cultivate character traits and qualities such as discipline, focus, and equanimity.

My thoughts and feelings were revolving more and more around loved ones, and how I was looking forward to sharing my appreciation, kindness, and love for them. This was quite amazing upon reflection, considering I was not at all close to family only one year ago.

My perceptions around love were incredibly distorted, which affected my way to give and receive it my entire life. With the help of the plant medicines, I've been able to reframe perspectives, open my heart, and change deep-seated behavioral patterns. I truly owe it to these sacred teacher plants for transforming my life for the better.

A greater sense of appreciation and gratitude was forming in more ways than one. I was remembering how important and grounding it was for me to spend even more time in nature. Feeling the cool crisp wind against my skin, smelling the fresh pine pollen, watching the birds flitter in and out between flowers and trees, embracing their chirps as they serenaded me with their songs. It made such a profound difference to the quality of my life.

Abstinence from human contact and communication, which was a great challenge for me, had surprisingly given me a deeper appreciation for silence, serenity, and the stillness within myself. The practice of removing verbal communication allowed me to fine tune my ability to hear and listen, not just in an auditory sense, but on a deeper observational level both internally and externally.

My shaman mentioned that she could see me soften in my face and my smile. I could feel it within. It was as if the hardened shell that formed around my heart was cracking open. When I nurtured the wounded/healing boy within, I could step into the space of being the man I wanted to become.

It seemed there were always layers to this, and I was constantly being given opportunities to come back to my integrity, back to my highest virtues, back to my softened and open heart.

Sigh. Another ceremony of not being able to fully surrender due to my concerns around breathing.

Shortly after the beginning of the Icaros, I left the room again so I wouldn't disturb others' journeys. I had the extremely distracting urge to expand my lungs to full capacity, forcefully coughing to try and dislodge anything in there. Although the medicine was having an influence on this, most of the unpleasantness was self-inflicted.

My lungs got a severe work over. I could feel how coarse they were, seemingly full of liquid, yet dry as a sponge at the same time. My body felt run down, with some sort of sinus infection accompanying my runny and blocked nose. It was so difficult finding the stillness within and letting go of control when my anchor point of steady calm breaths wasn't solid enough to fall back on.

The visual distortions were apparent in the bathroom. I watched the patterns on the floor breathe and gently swirl around, as I repeatedly coughed and spat in my bucket.

I ventured outside and listened to the chorus of frogs in the cool crisp air. I wasn't sure if the cold air was more of a detriment to my lungs, but being outside in the dark under the blanket of stars of the Milky Way galaxy was very grounding.

One of my shamans came outside. Sensing my discomfort, she presented a challenge to me. "Let go of your lungs," she whispered to me. "Let go of this story holding you back. Your lungs have been working hard. They're tired of carrying around this story…"

She blew mapacho smoke over me, and with some sweeping motions across my chest – which I understood to be clearing the energy surrounding my lungs – she disappeared back inside, leaving me to ponder this challenge she had offered.

After deep contemplation and much reflection, I began to

unravel what my shaman had shared.

Since my early childhood, I've carried the story of being an asthmatic; relying on daily asthma medications to stabilize respiratory function. This was true even more so when I suffered from unknown health issues travelling through the jungles, forests, volcanoes, reef systems, and coastline of Central America and the Caribbean.

Both infectious disease and liver specialists in Australia couldn't pinpoint why my liver enzymes were extremely elevated, which coincided with a weakened immune system – in particular, my poor respiratory function. Over the course of a year, my health slowly improved on its own, but since then, it was never quite the same.

Fast forward to my initial journey to the Amazon to work with the plant medicines, where I stopped taking asthma medications for an extended period – the first time I'd ever done so. It was only until a few months prior to La Dieta, that I was beginning to feel extremely run down and short of breath, so I resumed asthma medication for peace of mind.

The story I told myself from my past was that I've always had lung issues. Based on this story, I've held expectations of how I want my lungs to be. I've become attached to this old story of diminished health that no longer serves me. I grew attached to the desire of wishing for something else, while clinging to the past.

I needed a new narrative to release the old story and create something new. Of course, the past can be important in teaching us lessons and offering insight, yet I could see how holding onto this story was holding me back. I would get locked into the mindset that I know my body and I know my limits – based on past stories and experiences – but all this did was sabotage my ability to push beyond boundaries and explore what I was capable of. Whether it was purely a psychological attachment that I could release – asthma experts state that a lot of cases are psychological in nature – or something in my physiology and lifestyle that I needed to address, what I truly needed to do was surrender into complete acceptance of what is and rewrite my narrative.

What would a lifestyle of adhering to my highest principles and promoting optimal health and wellness look like? In pondering that thought, it all felt like such a risk: willingly putting myself into an altered state of consciousness, crossing my fingers for physical and psychological healing, but not knowing if I was going to have a respiratory malfunction, have my airways constrict, not be able to safely use any medication, and potentially take my last breath. Yet there was the great riddle of consciousness and the mystery of life itself. It's a miracle that we even exist at all and it's all transient. Nothing lasts forever.

So, could I become comfortable and accepting that I will have to take my last breath at some stage, potentially during ceremony?

Could I trust that my body would know what to do to look after itself, without my mind interjecting?

Could I at least pretend that all was fine, and surrender into illusory peace and stillness?

Could I trust that the medicine would truly help me heal?

Could I trust that my spirit was strong, and if necessary, could fight for the will to live?

Yet could I also trust that if it were truly my time to go, it would be my time to go?

Before ceremony, it was suggested that we build an altar in the garden, sit before it, and smoke some mapacho – sacred tobacco – to connect with the spirit of our master plant and ask for guidance with our intentions. I could feel the vibrational pulse within when I asked mapacho to deepen my connection to Chiric Sanango.

Going into ceremony, it was as if Chiric Sanango was piecing together my armor of courage, strength, integrity, discipline, and direction, while keeping my softened, vulnerable, loving, and compassionate heart contained within.

Distracting thoughts and feelings would try to creep in: What if it comes on too strong? What if it's terrifying? I can't wait for this to be over. Am I breathing okay? Do I need to cough or clear phlegm? Do I need a drink of water? But before I'd even finished these thought processes, they were met with a very stern "shh!" as if I was karate chopping these thoughts away with my mind before they had the chance to solidify. It seemed that my master plant, my new plant ally, was allowing me to channel higher levels of discipline and focus, and continuously helped straighten me back on track with the slightest awareness of distraction.

I was present. I was calm. I was ready.

With only a small cup of Ayahuasca, the medicine kicked in strong, and I experienced humbling, mind-blowing dimensions, full of wonderment and wisdom. Large humanoid beings made of twisting spirals gently greeted me into their world. Luminous grey twirling stripes were the undertone, while beautifully vibrant pastel colors flowed throughout. A white essence was the backdrop from which everything stemmed, signifying that this place was pure – a place for gentle healing.

These entities moved softly, caressing the space in which they carried themselves. We travelled through various landscapes, and with their elongated limbs, they produced glowing orbs which were presented to me as gifts of wisdom. I felt the wisdom of absolute trust in the medicine, the wisdom of trust that my body was fine, my body was strong, my body was okay to look after itself while I journeyed through these realms, and the deep wisdom of peace, stillness and oneness, once resistance was released and absolute surrender was embraced.

I had visions of gazing into a gigantic wooden vessel. The boards were running horizontal in the far distance, rising high into the sky; subtle blue tones made up the open ceiling. Inside this vast vessel were plants, trees, ferns and flowers, all lining the banks of a peaceful stream, which rose up into the highlands of the ship-like enclosure, disappearing into waterfalls and dense, scintillating, tropical vegetation. It was like I had stepped into the movie Avatar, a visionary utopia. It was breathtaking. My words always fall short of articulating these visions with much justice or accuracy.

Themes of loved ones appeared, as I opened my heart to family. Uncomfortable feelings accompanied these themes, and a purge ensued, which I understood to be the continued clearing of emotional baggage surrounding family, out with the old, in with the new. Getting rid of the negative connotations to make room for more love.

At some stage, Ayahuasca's realm shifted from luminous bright whites to a darker more sinister tone. I proceeded with caution. Slithering black circles rotated around, embedded with tantalizing gemstones that gave the impression of forbidden fruit. It felt as if a malevolent force was trying to hypnotize me, but this soon vanished as the medicine wore off.

I was deeply humbled and full of gratitude. I'd just received and embodied so much deep wisdom and teaching and I knew I was able to saddle up for another cup to test my strength, courage, and discipline to journey a little longer. There was no guarantee my experience would be pleasant again, but I called on the power of Chiric Sanango and crawled up to the altar in the darkness, sitting before my shamans.

There was more resistance after drinking again, yet time after time I kept allowing myself to drop into stillness. I was navigating an interesting world of fractal patterns when I was called on to share a prayer/blessing/song during ceremony. I wanted to decline, but somehow channeled some strength and cleared my throat. I allowed the medicine to pull, twist and contort my voice from deep inside me; a powerful Native American tone emerged as I chanted along. It was incredibly healing allowing that level of expression in such a vulnerable state in front of others journeying with Ayahuasca. It was a powerful form of solidifying one's sense of empowerment, voice, and expression in the world. Throughout the journey, Ayahuasca would let me know when it was time to purge, or clear my throat – without my mind's distractions or input from ego playing a part. There were moments it felt like I couldn't breathe when I needed to cough or purge, but still, I trusted my body, the medicine, and the process, and stayed true to the stillness within.

This is the most amazing part of all: by the end of the ceremony, I could breathe! My lungs didn't feel like a dry sponge, and it didn't feel like they were full of liquid. It was the clearest I had felt throughout the entirety of La Dieta, and for quite some time before that as well. My cold had diminished, and I felt strong and healthy. It was truly amazing. I sat there contemplating the scientific mechanisms at play to explain what was happening on the level of physical healing. It was difficult for me to comprehend. It felt as if the medicine collected old mucous from the crevasses and cavities in my lungs, pooled it together into a globular form, and allowed me to cough it all out.

It seemed like some kind of mechanism was being activated that allowed conditions preventing homeostasis in the body to be targeted and worked on by internal healing processes.

Whatever the explanation might be, the relationship that this medicine and the human body had, and the way they worked together so synergistically to provide multi-layered healing was nothing short of astounding. The further I journeyed and the more I drank the medicine, it became more and more clear that this was not just a psychedelic consciousness altering substance. There was something very mysterious at play, and I experienced it first hand on deeper and deeper levels each time I sat to drink. At the end of this journey, we eventually broke our diet with a delicious feast and communicated with the other Dieteros in a sharing circle. Before this, there was still ample time to process and reflect. There were many moments where the completion of this journey seemed so far away, yet by the end, it all went by in the blink of an eye; like it was all some sort of waking dream. Did all of it really just happen? It was bittersweet, as it always was finishing another cycle of work with the medicine.

It had become clear at this stage, that the core of this journey was about my health, and the process of releasing resistance into absolute surrender and stillness. In hindsight, I had many opportunities to become much more present throughout this odyssey, yet I also realized that it was the exact path that I needed to take to get me where I am currently sitting.

There were many things that I was bringing back with me: resilience of spirit and an armored plate of strength, discipline, integrity and direction. The softening of my heart, giving way to more compassion, kindness and love. Deeper trust in the medicine and my body. A renewed relationship with my health, and how I perceive it. Clarity and alignment with my highest virtues, values, health and wellness, and spirit. The wisdom of letting go of resistance into complete surrender. New appreciation and gratitude for serenity, silence and the stillness within. Re-connection with being outside in nature. Even more wonderment towards the magic of the medicine. Great preparation for my following weeks, returning to the Amazon Jungle. The question I found myself asking was how do I reintegrate and make sure these lessons and teachings stay with me?

In the past, I would ponder how I might act and what my behaviors might be like interacting in interpersonal relationships. Now, I feel I'm in a place where I don't need to project into the future and think about how I'm going to be, for the more I think about how I'm going to be, the less I'm actually being in the present moment. Like my dear medicine sister Nicole shared with me prior to La Dieta: "Don't try to be. Just be"

I trust I'll remember and embody the wisdom I've gained, and I'm certain over time that I'll momentarily forget, but that's what reintegration is all about for me: cultivating the practices in daily life that allow the alignment and authenticity of my deeper wisdom and truth to shine through.

Further reinforcement has become apparent that this is my master key. At least for now, the plant medicines are my ultimate tool of choice to help carve this inner path of self-mastery. It's a trial by fire and can be incredibly uncomfortable and challenging on many levels, yet for me it continues to keep unlocking and revisiting those deeper layers of inner wisdom, regarding my virtues, values, heart, and spirit.

I feel I'm in a great place for my second adventure back to Peru to work with the medicine. I've placed my foot on the first stepping stone, ready to further uncover and delve into more of the mysteries of the Universe, hopefully gaining more clarity, healing and wisdom along the way.

I am so grateful. I am so humbled.

Para el bien de todos.

For the good of all.

Gracias.

# THE ANCIENT FOREST

## Ayahuasca

I was just 19 years old and it was about a year after I had graduated high school. A friend that I had met in college told me that he was selling some Golden Teacher mushrooms, which are one of the most potent strains of mushrooms next to the Penis Envy strain, and they are not that easy to come by. Given the opportunity, I bought 5 grams the next day. I told my really good friend Alik that I had hit the goldmine with this and we planned a date to split them three weeks later.

Before I knew it, the night before the day we were going to do it had arrived. So many emotions ran through my mind that night: anxiety, excitement, and wonder. I wound up not falling asleep until about 4 a.m. I woke up around nine o'clock that morning and as I took a shower, I just kept thinking about how wild the day ahead of me was going to be. I ate some waffles completely plain because when I have anxiety my stomach can barely hold anything down and it was the only thing I seemed to be able to eat.

It was around 10 a.m. and Alik was running late, which led me to nervously pace around my house for an hour awaiting his arrival. When he finally arrived, we wasted no time. I had already split the mushrooms into 2.5 grams each. We walked across the street to a small section of woods that separated my street from the highway. We opened the small  sandwich bags I had put them in and ate them as fast as we possibly could. The taste was horrible. I was barely able to chew them before I swallowed every cap and stem.

We were planning on waiting for my friend Bryan to arrive and drive us to a spot that was more suitable for tripping. Bryan had heard that we were going to trip and wanted to be there. He had told us that he liked being in the presence of people that were tripping, however, Bryan was running late so we decided to walk and just meet him at the spot.

The walk was about 1.5 miles long and about halfway through the walk I had already started to notice a subtle impact from the mushrooms. I looked over at Alik and we both smiled. Nothing was really said, but we were both on the same page; the mushrooms were starting to kick in. The subtle impact was followed by a large amount of unpleasantness in my stomach. It was only about twenty to twenty-five minutes in and I was already fighting the urge to throw up. My stomach is notorious for not being able to process anything, so this didn't surprise me. I just didn't want to throw up so soon and risk not absorbing all of the Psilocybin.

We were about five hundred feet from our destination when the trip really started to kick in for me. I was walking next to very tall grass and a piece was right out in front of me, so I stuck my hand out and let the piece of grass slide through my fingers. As soon as I did that it felt like I had just jumped through a wormhole. My vision became so crisp and clear, I started to notice all of the bugs that were flying around. Green never looked so green to me, and blue never looked so blue to me.

My hearing slowed down and I started to pick up on noises that were always happening in the background, but I had always seemed to tune out. My sense of time started to really slow down at this point. It started to look and sound like everything was happening in slow motion. Slow motion was something that was always prevalent in all of my trips, and it was one of the only things that seemed to freak me out a little bit. Something about my sense of time being messed with gave me anxiety, but when the trip progressed I got more and more comfortable with the change in perception.

Finally, we arrived at our destination, an abandoned football field with a bunch of trails in the back where a lot of people would ride dirt bikes. Bryan arrived at the same exact time we did. Alik and I weren't saying much and we both kind of telepathically knew that both of our stomachs were feeling extremely unwell. My mind was racing at this point as I was getting adjusted to this new state of consciousness. I was thinking that Alik and I were both in for a bad trip.

After sitting for a couple of minutes, we watched the trees breathe and soon decided that it would be best if we took a walk into the woods to see if our stomachs would get better. Before we could even make it to the beginning of the trail I threw up. I remember being extremely paranoid at this moment because cars could still come in and see us, and I didn't want to deal with anyone wondering why I was throwing up. As I threw up I could feel all the unchewed caps burst out of my mouth, as well as the plain waffles that I had that morning. Bryan was patting my back in an effort to comfort me, which oddly enough seemed to help a lot. I got the first purge over with but my stomach was still not right. We walked for another five minutes and boom, I had to throw up again. This time I was a lot less paranoid about throwing up, but I still remember feeling extremely vulnerable as I puked because throwing up isn't exactly the "toughest" thing a guy can do.

At this point, the intensity of the trip had drastically increased. The hardest part of throwing up was when I closed my eyes. A powerful image of what I can only describe as a Godhead appeared in my mind whenever I closed my eyes to throw up. This provoked indescribable emotions in me. As soon as I finish throwing up I looked over and Alik began to purge as well. Bryan was just standing there waiting for us to keep moving. There was just an unspoken respect for each other and there was no fuss about us throwing up.

After Alik finished throwing up we continued our trek through the woods. I stared at the ground the entire time we were walking; the patterns in the ground were so beautiful and complex. They looked as if they were always there but I could never notice them until now. After throwing up, I was finally starting to get a lot more comfortable with the trip. I stopped fighting the trip and started to ride it instead.

After about ten or so minutes of walking we made it to the top of a decently sized hill where there was a bunch of sand. Alik and I decided to take a break here because the mushrooms were giving us a stony body high that was wearing us both out a little bit.

I stood at the top of the hill and looked at everything below me. Everything seemed so tranquil and peaceful. The birds and the crickets were chirping and a slight breeze blew in the trees. All of my worries from before the trip had faded and this ineffable joy had overcome me. A sense of oneness started to take hold. The microcosm and the macrocosm felt like they were bleeding together to create the masterpiece that was being observed by my consciousness.

Alik kicked off his shoes and started doing somersaults, which led me to kick off my shoes and enjoy the sand beneath my toes.

We decided that we wanted to go further into the woods. We left our shoes at the top of the hill and walked onto a different trail, both of us still barefoot. A strange vibration came over me when we stepped into the trails. It felt like I had jumped back in time. All of the trees and plants were giving off an ancient feeling. It wasn't long before I stepped on a piece of glass and got really freaked out. Alik noticed the heavy vibration that I had just caught and we decided to turn around. The glass felt symbolic for something and it made me begin to think about the destruction of Earth that is happening at the hands of humans and how much healthier the planet was during ancient civilizations.

When we arrived back at the top of the hill I decided to take a seat and just breathe. I looked over at Alik and could see his aura. It was bright red and it gave off a very euphoric feeling. Prior to this I had never seen anyone's aura before, as LSD had failed to provoke this in me.

After sitting in silence for a good amount of time, we

decided to head back to the entrance of the abandoned football field. My head was in the clouds at this point and I really don't remember much about the walk back. When we finally got there, I started pacing back and forth around Bryan's car. Being in a place where anyone could pull in was making me a little uncomfortable. As I was pacing, I caught my reflection in the window of Bryan's car. Looking at myself while peaking on mushrooms was pretty insane to say the least. My eyes were as wide as an owl's, and there was this evil looking smirk on my face. My face looked animated and it seemed like I was glowing.

Bryan suggested that we go to the store to pick up something to drink and that he would drive us. I hopped in the front seat and Alik hopped in the back. As we were driving to the store, I kept having this feeling that something malevolent was happening to the world. I was thinking about all of the things that I had been reading about the state of the world and how it was personally impacting me at this very moment. The thoughts were really freaking me out so I tried my best to get a hold of them.

This five minute drive to the store finally came to end even though it felt much longer. As soon as I got out of the car I fell. The mushroom body high was in full force. I caught myself on my right hand before I fell and I quickly got up. As soon as I got up a cop car was driving by. I was extremely relieved that he didn't see that. The police in my town find everything suspicious, which always kept me on my toes and made me develop a paranoid mindset even when I was sober. I looked at my hand and there was a tiny cut, nothing serious, but the pattern it made was enough to intrigue me.

We all walked into the store and picked up something to drink and then headed back to my house. I was still way too high to go into my house so I suggested that Bryan drive Alik's car to the beach. It was still pretty early in the day and we needed something to do to kill some time, plus I figured the beach would be awesome on mushrooms.

Bryan and Alik both agreed and we were off. We stopped at another convenience store to pick up some more snacks and drinks before we drove all the way there. When we made it to the register, the cashier was looking at us funny and asked if she knew Alik. This interaction was making me very nervous. Even the simplest of things can change your mindset when you're in the midst of a trip. Luckily she had nothing to say to me and I bought my stuff and walked back to Alik's car where Bryan was waiting for us.

We hopped on the highway and started heading to the beach. I was sitting in the back seat and played music off of my phone. Every song sounded so beautiful. I was dancing and singing and for the first time I truly knew what catharsis was. I felt so free and uninhibited.

At a certain point during the drive, I decided to lay down since I had the whole back seat to myself. As I was laying down, we drove through a rainstorm. I started to think about the end of my first real relationship and how even though it was a couple of years ago I was still not fully over it. The rain was synchronizing so well with the emotional moment that I was having. After a couple of miles, the rainstorm was over and the sun was shining again. I now had this new understanding of how sunshine wouldn't feel so good if it wasn't for rain and how joy wouldn't feel so good if it wasn't for pain. I finally felt like I had some closure on the relationship.

As I looked out the window I felt so connected with the Earth, Alik, and Bryan. I remember having this overwhelming feeling of love for them. I wanted badly to just say "I love you guys" but the moment didn't seem right since the music was still blasting.

After about an hour we finally arrived at the beach and found parking. At this point the trip was starting to level off. Everything was still really bright and beautiful, but the patterns were starting to fade. The beach was the perfect place for us to come down. About four and a half hours had passed since we first ate the mushrooms. Alik ran into the water and went for a quick swim while Bryan and I walked up the beach. Bryan told me some stuff that he wanted to get off his chest and I happily listened and gave him advice to the best of my ability. We only stayed at the beach for about a half hour before we decided to leave.

About twenty minutes into the drive home I had pretty much fully come down. The experience was so powerful though. I felt so renewed and refreshed after the trip was over.

All in all, psychedelics have made a huge long-lasting impact on my life. They can truly be used for transformative purposes. If they're used with care and respect they can become amazing tools for self-reflection, self-growth, and can help you reach a better understanding of yourself and the world around you. The walls between yourself, others, and the environment are broken down to show the interconnectedness between everything that exists.

# DISSOLVING THE ILLUSION

## LSD

Since the day that I could coalesce a conscious inner voice, I have felt as though the expanse of the human experience is being shrouded in an illusion of limitation. Limitation to this reality and to the eighty or so some years of experience we have here. Where did this illusion originate and what was the truth on the other side? This was something I couldn't understand until the illusion was dissolved.

This was the day my life changed forever. The prior morning, I had received a text from my best friend Trevor asking if I wanted to do LSD with him for the first time. Keep in mind this was my first ever psychedelic experience. He, on the other hand, had been through a few trips before. Our plan was to wake up at the crack of dawn, drive the hour and a half to our buddy's cottage on Lake Michigan in Door County, Wisconsin, take the LSD, and then play it by ear from there… and so we did.

We arrived at the cottage around 8 a.m. on what must have been the most picturesque day of summer to date. I took one tab of the LSD and Trevor took two, after which we proceeded to smoke a morning bowl with our friend before he headed off to work. Before leaving he gave us the okay to use his kayaks if we felt so inclined, much to our delight. It wasn't more than twenty minutes after our friend had left that we began to feel the early effects of the LSD.

As we sat discussing our next move we both fell silent. I felt the energy of the room was disturbed by what I can only explain as the feeling of slowly fleeing life. My eyes locked on a vase of wilting flowers in the middle of the table. I stared, turned to my friend, and exclaimed, "Those flowers are so sad. They're dying, right now, right here." Not a single exchange of words was spoken after that statement, as we both stood and replaced the water in the vase and carefully placed the flowers outside in the sun. Just as fast as the feelings of impending death had overwhelmed us, the energies of life, empathy, and oneness took its place. Standing with feelings of accomplishment, and love, and a grin from ear to ear, we moved onward.

As we began brainstorming our official game plan, it soon came to us. We decided to take the kayaks and paddle to an island a few miles off the shore of Lake Michigan. Packing our bags and getting the boats launched were aggravatingly tedious tasks. Each push onward to achieve any kind of progress was quickly halted by moments of awe and an ever-loosening grip of our egos, only to realize zero progress had been made. Despite falling into a slight purgatory, we managed to get on the water and on with our day; and what a day it was. I had never felt so free, so alive. As the bow of the kayak cut through the waves I was showered with what seemed like the most purely divine droplets of water I had ever experienced. They underwent a sort of mitosis in midair, traveled in slow motion and then found their way to my skin where their mere presence manifested the most indescribable feeling. Never in my life had I experienced water in such a way.

Like clockwork, our already heightened pace increased in what seemed like a feat of superhuman proportions. The stamina was unlike anything I had ever seen. At one point, we had so much speed that we were actually able to catch and ride the wake of the yachts and shipping boats passing by.

Like a green, timeless turtle shell, the island emerged from the skyline and grew closer with every stroke of our paddles. The homogeneous blue depths of Lake Michigan gave way to a rocky bottom that gently loosened its grip from the cold waters… we were there. Out of our boats, we hugged and jumped in a display of unrelenting happiness and bliss. It felt as though we took the place of ancient explorers lost at sea who had just found their only hope for survival. Here we hung up our hammocks, ate our subs, and attempted to roll a joint the best we could considering our states. After a failed attempt that resulted in a picture-perfect joint, albeit the size of a thumbtack, we rolled up again and set off to hike the island.

As we strolled about, our minds willingly slipped and unhinged into a world entirely its own. The trees hummed in exchanging and complimentary frequencies. The waves crashed on the shore and echoed into what felt like eternity. After some time, neither of us fully knew why, but it was time to go. We had nowhere to be, no other plans, but it was time to go. Just as we had come, we had left, off the shore, through the churning waters of Lake Michigan and into the calm bay of our friend's cottage.

What is the happiest moment in your life? I mean truly

happy. This exact moment was it for me. The exact moment we drifted over the glass like water of the bay and returned home. It was as if the hand of the Universe had its grip on my soul. I lay back in the kayak with my eyes closed and was overwhelmed with an incomprehensible amount of pure unadulterated love, compassion, empathy, and source energy. I was fully unfastened from my physical form: no more attachment, no more suffering, no more regret of the past and anxiety of the next moment. I simply just... was. It was then that I knew that this was the true me. This was the state of being to strive and maintain in life regardless of psychedelic intake.

After taking a load off in the living room, we set off again, but this time on a hike through town and into Peninsula State Park. The town was a small, cozy lakeside town that soon took on the likeness of a child's plastic town playset. Cars, buildings, people, and clouds all appeared to be ripped directly from the toy aisle. The flowers had looked like the plastic flower humming bird feeders in my grandmother's backyard. As we passed the busy beach in a mesmerized state of wonder, I became overwhelmed by a wall of energy. It was as if my brain was acting as a type of antenna and I was picking up everybody's presence on the beach. It was very reminiscent of the feeling you get when you think someone is following you, only amplified by a factor of ten. I very easily could have let this wave of energy overtake me, but I stood fast. I simply acknowledged its existence and moved on.

It was at this point that we had begun our descent from the LSD induced spiritual play land and entered the mystic woods of Peninsula State Park. We figured it was only appropriate to find a spot we could ride out the end of our trip; preferably in our hammocks of course. As the Law of Attraction would have it, we came across a forty-foot cliff perfect for climbing. It was certainly not the most difficult climb we had attempted. Atop was a patch of old growth oak trees from which we planned to hang our hammocks and end our day.

My friend began his ascent first, as he had always been a full-speed-ahead kind of guy. Shortly after, I followed with great ambition. Foot, hand, foot, hand, and so on. Sweat built up on my brow until it gave way like a broken water dam trickling down the contour of my face. My breaths synchronized with the rock face in front of me and the forest floor slowly fell away. An ambiance of tranquility was abruptly halted by a wave of infinitesimal sadness. It was as if every particle of happiness and security were being sucked from my soul. My breathing became erratic, cold sweats began their icy grip over my body, and I felt myself struggling to stay on the edge of consciousness as my bare hands and feet dug deep into the cliff side. The sound of rocks dislodging from their ancient tombs and shattering on the floor below echoed with taunting danger.

Although severely shaken and with no end to this torture in sight, I knew my only chance to make it out okay was to keep climbing. With my eyes shut and breathing controlled to the best of my ability, I said to myself, "You are here, you are present, and you are powerful." My eyes opened with raw determination and confidence as I peered up at the last fifteen feet to the top. The more progress I made, the better I felt. I climbed faster and faster until... I had done it. It was over.

I lied motionless on my back with my legs still hanging off the edge in a hyperventilating heap of exhaustion. The water painted canopy of the old growth trees above danced in the wind, letting beams of the most iridescent sunlight warm my battle worn soul. The biggest smile crept across my face as I began to cry with happiness and accomplishment. As I discreetly wiped my tears and took a deep breath, my friend, who was oblivious to the whole ordeal, turned around with his hammock half set up and said, "Thanks for coming on this adventure with me man, love you brother." I smiled, stood, and walked over to begin setting up my hammock.

Here we spent the last two hours of our trip. The forest below gave way to the vast deep blue of Lake Michigan. sunlight danced off the leaves, refracting into my eyes and creating a kaleidoscopic mosaic that seemed to move on command as I reached out with my fingertips to touch them. We swung at the mercy of the breeze and watched as the last hours of an unforgettable day slowly came to an end.

So here we are; what are we left with? We're left with a young man forever transformed in a way he had yet to understand. All he knew was that it was for the better. This transcendental movie frame of experience added to the reel of his life was one that would set in motion a vortex of spiritually heightening events beyond all he could have ever imagined.

As days, weeks, months, and years passed, the seeds of consciousness planted that beautiful summer day long ago had blossomed into realizations of unspeakable humility and virtue.

He now understood the true power of love, the existence of universal oneness, and that each individual was a beautifully unique conscious expression of the Universe acting as a mirror for the whole of the Universe to experience itself. He recognized that within this 3D flesh-suit we carry around day after day, resides a holographic fractal of infinite consciousness, knowledge, and source energy that is currently having one out of an infinite number of experiences coalesced from the nursery crib of possibilities – a pure everlasting beam of light and love that is capable of transcending all time, space, and dimensions. When the time comes to part from this 3D physical plane of existence and your flesh-suit begins to degrade, fear not eternal nothingness, but instead embrace the transcendence of your consciousness and open up to the next chapter of experience.

# THE CRYSTAL TOWERS

## DMT

"You a divine being. You matter, you count. You come from realms of unimaginable power and light, and you will return to those realms." -Terence McKenna

Ernest Hemingway once wrote, "Writing is architecture, not interior design." As a writer, the most effective strategy in creating magic is being able to discover it. To create stories, characters, scenes, music, lighting, we must imagine universes of our own making from within. Writing comes from within, and since writing is the magic, DMT was the magician. It opened the doorway to a strange and fascinating world and my acquaintance with that world elevated my imagination.

A friend of mine helped to make this dream a reality. He invited me over to his apartment to blast me off. I was excited and remarkably nervous about trying this particular psychedelic, as I knew it had the power to give you an almost out of body experience.

I cleansed my body with a complete and total detox. No marijuana and no alcohol of any kind. It was the complete annihilation of negative energy and I wanted my mind to be a blank canvas. This proved to be most effective considering how exhilarating it felt to not be strapped down by these dependencies that help to alleviate life's stress. I prepared myself all day through meditation, reading, and getting plenty of exercise to help expedite the detoxification process. It was as if I were shedding my skin and ridding myself of old wounds, anger and bitterness – a removal from my former self.

I left my apartment, and as I drove to my friend's house all I kept thinking about was how real this situation was and how beautiful this reality was to me. It was the pivotal moment in my life where I knew the Universe heard my plea and in its infinite power made it happen. I never in a million years thought something of this magnitude would have made itself known, but it has and there is no time like the present. During the drive, I felt such inner peace. I was exactly where I needed to be on my path to enlightenment.

The roads were clear and the sky was dark with a shining omniscient moon. Music played with grace and fluidity as it steadied my anxiety about trying DMT for the first time. I met him and we had dinner, becoming acquainted with each other. After dinner, I was lucky enough to meet three friends of his. We exchanged stories about psychedelics and our experiences, perspectives, and tales of adventure and spiritual growth. He graciously gave me a crystal called black tourmaline, which is known for its ability to rid the atmosphere around you of negative energy, I was grateful to have it in my possession, as I did feel its magic in my hands.

After an hour or two, we drove back to his apartment. During my drive, I was able to get to get to know one of his friend's, as he told everything he knew about DMT and its potency on the human mind and body. We near my friend's apartment and as we walked, he told me to close my eyes and take three deep breaths. The air was cold, but gratification came in an awesome wave.

We walked inside, up the elevator, and into my friend's apartment. I sat down and complimented him on the beautiful apartment. He offered me some water and a calming drink that was a ceremonial sacrament in the South Pacific, almost like a liquid sedative, called Kava Kava. He fixed it up for me and within minutes my fears were gone. I laid down on this chair with my feet up with a giant blanket on me, as they told me I may get cold. I had a pair of sleeping shades to cover my eyes from all outside distractions. He told me to let him know when I was completely ready to smoke the DMT. This was it… my thrust into hyper-drive.

The lights were turned off and the only light was coming from the TV, as shamanic music was playing over the speakers. The image of a gorgeous blue sky with a colorful horizon over a tree that stood alone glowed in the dark. He informed me to take three deep pulls from the pipe that he filled with white crystals. He also told me to remember to breathe and most importantly, to surrender to the medicine. The feeling of resistance during the experience was only that of my ego, fighting to the end to resist its impending death. We also briefly discussed how Terence McKenna described it as smelling like "burning plastic" and he was right on the money – it was awful. He told me, "Whenever you're ready," waiting with a great calm to light it up. I told him one minute, as I sat in the comfortable chair with my legs up breathing in through my nose and out my mouth. I finally told him, "Yeah, I'm ready dude."

He sparked the lighter and held it toward the white looking crystals. I took a long hard pull from the pipe and immediately coughed it out. In no time, I was already feeling its heavy effects. I took another hit and coughed it out again. My friend advised me to take a smaller hit, and one last little puff was all it fucking took! All I remember saying before closing my eyes and surrendering to it was, "Oh shit, I'm definitely feeling it now." I was in!

I laid back and continued to breathe in through my nose and out through my mouth. It was so surreal. I felt like I was inside a giant ocean of color and sound. I had never felt such a rush of energy being blasted from my body and with such potency. It all happened with such an incomprehensible speed and felt like I was going two hundred miles an hour. It was as if it were channeling another universe with each deep breath. The chair seemed to move but it wasn't moving. It was like a force from some unknown presence had arrived inside my friend's living room and took me by the hand to lead me beyond the white horizon of my being.

I entered through a large oak door that stood over two-hundred feet tall into the infinite skyline. My hand lightly pressed against it and the doors slowly opened. Contrary to popular belief, it wasn't exactly enlightenment that I felt. It was realization. It was seeing everything that I'd ever done, said, and experienced, limitless and profound. After walking through the doors with rising trepidation, an invisible presence with its hand, led me over the threshold. What I saw galvanized me. It was an enormous green grid that had endless windows, and before I knew it, it became a rushing light flooding everything around it.

It wasn't about discovering the answer, it was about searching for the question. Now a majority of people had inquired about what I had been searching for by trying DMT and my response was always the same. That's what I'm hoping to find out. After seeing the inexplicable beauty and complexity of the giant green grid, it disappeared and the next chapter of my radiating DMT trip continued.

Next, I came across glowing red-orange eyes. It was in a puff of blue and red smoke that surrounded this mystical being's face, almost like a shroud. These eyes weren't evil, angry, dark, or foreboding but understanding. They had a mystery to them and possessed a great sense of wisdom and comfort in this magical world. They told me everything that I needed to know and whispered a great song to me that only I could hear. The eyes moved around the infinite space of stars and comets, of bursting noises, and symphonic colors, but they maintained their warm gaze as they passed through my solar plexus and rejuvenated my soul.

I started laughing quietly and then shed tears. Great warm memories of family members that had passed before me appeared and I couldn't breathe. They were all there sitting in front of me having wine and dinner. They had never felt as real to me as they did in that moment. It was like being embraced by a friend that you hadn't seen in ages, those loving and familiar affections that you only feel a few times throughout your life. This encounter resembled a lucid dream and they quickly disappeared.

Next, a city of glass appeared. Towers that were over three hundred feet tall and made of clear beautiful white crystal appeared in front of me in glowing white light. A giant blinding infinite light as bright as the sun stood above me in glorious color. I was flying among the towers, looking inside of them, seeing orbs and rays of light projecting life and energy into the towers' monolithic rooms. The color of each crystal glowed in yellow and white, with hints of blue and red, and they seemed to swirl around the towers like dancing fireworks. The atmosphere was warm, but not hot. It felt like the temperature of my own skin. I was realizing so much during my tour of the city of glass and it helped me to remember that the spiritual world is a real place, not just a beautiful idea.

I heard the wind through the clouds, the whistling birds, the chirping crickets, and saw the towers glistening an exploding light that we as human beings carry inside of us, giving hope to everyone and anything, but most importantly, to ourselves. I was Superman up there in the netherworld of my mind and doors were being kicked the fuck down, walls were being bulldozed, my ego was being shattered, and my heart was a symphony of drums. I was completely removed from my physical body as I broke through to the other side. As the towers disappeared, everything was white. Never before had I seen my own world with such heightened power and clarity, and in keeping with this newfound clarity, I will carry it with me for the rest of my life.

The last stage of this wonderful experience was a giant blue circle in front of my eyes that was breathing, morphing, and expanding. It was the epitome of my experience with DMT, the enriching psychedelic journey becoming a navigator of the infinite. The circle was enormous and it grew with each deep conscious breath, moving with unimaginable speed beyond the white horizon.

As the trip came to a gentle and swift conclusion, I opened my eyes and saw the blue light in front of me. It was around my friend who was waiting for my return. Right away he asked, "What did you think?" I felt a giant weight over me as if I couldn't even move. I was still, quiet, and content. "That was unbelievable," I said, as I laughed to myself. I kept remembering the images that had just unfolded before me and I vividly described it to my friends in the room. They were all eager to know what I thought and how it felt being blasted out of my body. The feeling alone is worth its weight in gold. As I spoke about my experience, they wondered if I had spoken to the entities that regularly appeared in the metaphysical DMT world. I responded, "No, but I felt like they were guiding me. What they showed me was their communication to me. That was their message. Their gifts were these realizations I had been given."

As amazing as it was to be a part of the spiritual world, or the "realms of light" as Terence McKenna called it, it was also exceedingly baffling to me on how elusive the experience was, and how after what seemed like hours was in fact was only twenty minutes.

I was myself again and all those memories and visions slowly disappeared. I knew I had to write it all down before they evaporated completely. I understood my obligation to my first DMT trip and I was committed to it. Centuries of wisdom in only twenty minutes, needless to say, and I'm still trying to understand this about DMT. These chances don't come around often, so when a chance of this magnitude presents itself you need to take full advantage of it no matter if you feel nerves, anxiety, or doubt. Those emotions are sustaining, but they are also transient and regret is permanent. Wisdom is and always will be the most valuable thing that you possess and nobody can take it from you.

Love comes in many forms, but none as glorious as the form of inner light. A light that can never go out. A light that you yourself can show to the world to cast out the darkness, push it over the edge and down the mountain. I remember the excitement I felt while discussing my experience. It was a journey, a wild, fast and unpredictable journey in another world. I remember *2001: A Space Odyssey's* last and final line in the film, "The four-million-year-old black monolith has remained completely inert. It's origin and purpose still a total mystery." That's how I perceived my acquaintance with DMT, never knowing the answer and being comfortable with that fact. I had discovered that answers aren't necessary when you are exploring your soul. What's necessary is an open mind and a beating heart. My trip was over, but my understanding of it had just begun.

# EARTH,
# THE GRAND STAGE

## LSD + MDMA

For months leading up to the experience, I couldn't understand why my friend wouldn't shut up about Burning Man. I would come to learn that until you experience it for yourself, you really have no idea. For years I had seen pictures of people at Burning Man and it seemed like a recreation of the world of post-apocalyptic Mad Max.. I was always intrigued, but the thought to actually take the plunge seldom entered my mind.

I had reconnected with a close childhood friend of mine who I had lost touch with. It was the longest we hadn't spoken since we met in the first grade. For me, it was always the most impulsive decisions that led to the most powerful eye-opening experiences, so when he extended the invitation to come to Burning Man, which took place during my 30th birthday, naturally I said "fuck it, I'm going." But I really had no idea what I was in for, how powerful this experience would truly be, or for how it would change me. I would soon understand what the fuss was all about.

I had been on my own transformative path leading up to my first "burn," as the veteran Burners call it, and this experience felt like it had been deliberately laid out before me. Like something knew I needed it and made sure I found my way there. And so, I went.

We flew into Reno and rented our RV, piled our stuff in and prepared our home away from home for the next week. On the way, we overheard that the desert had flooded from heavy rainfall and that the festival gates were closed, so we pulled off of the highway and rested for the night. After an exhausting 11-hour drive, we finally arrived.

Once the ancient lakebed of Lake Lahontan in the harsh Nevada desert, they called it "The Playa." The desert is a seriously unforgiving place, so leave it to humans to gather by the tens of thousands in the most inhospitable place for an uplifting experience. Although it now seems so appropriate looking back. It is only when we are pushed beyond our comfort – physically, mentally, and emotionally – and the familiarity of modern securities are removed that we truly learn who we are. Sleep deprivation. Hunger. Dehydration. Fatigue. These are common amongst Burners, but I came to accept them as an integral part of my experience, well outside of my comfort zone.

We arrived at our camp site and pulled the RV into our designated space. We were welcomed by our campmates, some more welcoming than others. Some of them would continue to be standoff-ish the entire week, while others treated us like family. Once we were all set up, we got dressed and prepared for our first night out.

We had purchased bicycles at a Wal Mart in Reno to prepare for the journey. The Playa covers several square miles, so traveling in the desert on foot is just a terrible idea. The only vehicles allowed to drive as a means of transportation were "art cars," which are essentially intricate and mind-bending works of art on wheels. Some even have high-powered audio equipment on them so a party can take place wherever they set down their anchor. But for us, and most others, bicycles would be a saving grace.

We rode out at first sundown and headed toward the center of The Playa where "The Man" stood. The Man was at the center of the Burning Man experience. Over fifty feet tall, and built bigger each year, The Man was a wooden effigy of a human, and at the end of the week, they burn The Man as a representation of many things. The burning of things that no longer serve us. The burning of the self. The ego. Our past. Our fears. The burning of anything that needs to be burned in order for us to grow and become our highest and truest self. There is something very primal and very sacred about fire. It is both a destroyer and a creator, and through that destruction, like a phoenix rising from the ashes, we are reborn more powerful than before. We have to die a thousand times to know who we are and more importantly who we are not.

As we approached on our bicycles, in the expanse between the camp sites and The Man, there were neon lights in every direction as far as the eye could see. Everyone and everything was lit up. It literally too my breath away. I had to stop riding to process this sensory overload. All I could think was "This is it. I had no idea." This would become a phrase that repeat itself throughout the week. The dust. The lights. It does something to you.

When we finally arrived at The Man, I looked up in awe. I looked at him as if I were looking at myself, anticipating its destruction. As I walked closer, I could see writing on the legs of The Man, as high as people's arms could reach. One thing stood out from the rest: *Love is the only infinite resource in the Universe.* A powerful idea, but life-changing once understood. Everyone around me was hugging, embracing one another. Most of them complete strangers. Everyone was ranting about being "home." Moments later, a total stranger walked up to me and said "Welcome home!" and gave me a big hug. Actually, it was more than a hug. It was an embrace. They embraced me as if they knew me all their life and hadn't seen me in years. As if it were the first and last time we would ever cross paths. And it was. This felt like a piece that was missing. Actually, one that we are all missing. We spend most of our lives in isolation from one another, afraid of real connection. We fear being hurt and live our lives in that perpetual state. What a strange world we live in. Imagine if everyone wasn't so guarded?

In that moment I felt so welcomed, so loved, and more importantly so accepted. This was revelatory for me. Above all, all we want is to be accepted, and in this acceptance you learn to accept yourself. In many ways, it is the fear that others do not accept you for who you are that can become the reason you do not accept yourself. It is a relentless and vicious cycle. One that most do not know they are even in. For me, this experience broke down those walls.

It was not until the second night that I had indulged in psychedelics. I had tripped a lot in my youth, but a few bad mushroom trips derailed me. For years, I had carried this ever-growing fear that I could never *not* have a "bad" trip again. This fear became a monster that I let define me. Just prior to Burning Man I had a close friend of mine follow me into the woods to help guide me through a mild LSD experience, specifically so I could break this cycle, regain my footing, and overcome my fear. I desperately wanted to take LSD at Burning Man and I was convinced that this had to happen in order for me to not be afraid. So I took half a tab and surrendered to the experience. It was mild, but it was enough for me to know that I could be free of bad trips if I just trusted the medicine and entered the experience without fear and without expectation. I was ready.

The second night at Burning Man had arrived and I was mentally prepared for what was ahead. I took 200 mg of pure MDMA along with one tab of LSD and waited in anticipation. We rode around the desert on our bicycles and explored all of the sights and sounds and there were moments where I had completely forgotten I had taken anything, until the familiar and warm sensations of MDMA kicked in. Slowly, all of my inhibitions, about myself and others, dissipated into the desert night. Riding through the desert under the star-filled sky felt like we were kids again, space bandits riding on the Moon.

We gravitated toward whatever called us and eventually found our way back to the RV to get more water and take a break from the noise. When we entered the RV, it seemed like such an alien place. It was filled with things that were once familiar, but I couldn't quite remember what they were or where they came from. We gathered our things and left the RV to explore the desert once again, but my friend asked me to get something from the RV. Once I entered the RV, the LSD was kicking hard and I found myself having to become reacquainted with very basic and simple things. This simple task became a massive undertaking, and what normally took moments to accomplish now took forever. My memory would lapse and I would have to remember not just the task at hand, but the entire chain of events that led up to that task. I looked at my hands and didn't understand what they were, let alone that they belonged to me. It was as if I had returned to my infancy, having to relearn everything about who I was, what I was, how things operated and how they were related to one another. I was looking at everything for the first time again. This was disorienting to say the least and my ability to communicate with others and "be human" would continue to deteriorate. Probably better off that I was alone for some of these experiences because I probably looked like a complete maniac. But I was content in my confusion and I continued figuring out why I was in the RV.

I got lost inside the RV for god knows how long and eventually stumbled into the bathroom. As I entered, I turned to the mirror and looked at myself. My pupils were so wide that I couldn't see the color of my iris. I got lost in my reflection, until my reflection came to life. The mirror image of myself became its own being with its own identity. It observed me as I observed it. It spoke to me and said, "You are a good man with a big heart. Don't ever forget that. You are a vessel for something greater." Looking back, I still wonder if this was just me talking to myself, but I was so engulfed in that moment that I lost all sense of self and listened to my own advice objectively.

This man in the mirror knew that I had been hurt in a

thousand ways and how I never understood why. He knew I had been distrusting, selfish, and a careless with my decisions. He knew that I repeated the same mistakes over and over again and hurt so many people along the way. He watched me beat myself up for these mistakes day in and day out, and that my internal conflict was like a poison slowly killing me inside. He saw how I was angry at the world for all of its flaws and frustrated because I didn't understand why people were so fucking bad to one another. He saw that I was confused. He saw my suffering. He saw how I felt lost. But in that moment, the man in the mirror looked back at me and we locked eyes. His eyes told me everything. The man in the mirror looked at me with love and acceptance. I was lost in the gaze of his eyes as they told me that everything would be okay. I was mesmerized. His eyes told me to trust in myself and more importantly to trust in my heart. His eyes told me to let go of who "I" was and to let go of my "story" that I had allowed to not only define me, but to become me. I hadn't realized until that moment that I could perceive myself objectively and see my past fuck ups as a different person, and not "me," but a different version of me and not who I am today. His eyes told me, without words, that I could finally breathe. I am human and it is okay. My flaws were not a weakness of mine, nor were they a sign of failure. They are a natural part of the human process and should be looked at without judgment. We are here to fuck up, and we are here to learn. It is *why* we are here.

I parted ways with the man in the mirror, and I felt different. I felt lighter. I left that RV accepting myself for the very first time. Something changed in me during that exchange in the

Some long-awaited switches were finally turned on and off, and I could feel it.

I left the RV and returned to the desert night. Feeling empowered, I dosed some more MDMA and took another tab of LSD, ready for the journey ahead. We rode around as a group under an ocean of stars. As I was riding, I looked to my right and saw ancient structures out in the desert reminiscient of Egyptian pyramids and monoliths, covered in inscriptions. These structures faded in and out of my perception and there were a few moments where I got a good look at them. It felt less like a visual hallucination and more like I was getting a glimpse into a very ancient past. Eventually these structures faded out and I continued riding along smiling, in awe of what I had just seen.

We arrived at Robot Heart, arguably one of the most incredible performances on The Playa, but I was too loaded to dance. I was out of my mind and wanted to be alone. We parked our bikes and everyone walked into the crowd as I stayed behind. I stood by the bikes and laid down in the dust by myself. I lit up a cigarette and watched the smoke rise up toward the stars, shifting and morphing. I was lost in myself.

As I laid there, I could hear the sounds of joy emanating from the interactions around me. The MDMA gently took hold of me and I was overcome by this complete euphoria, connected to everything around me. I could literally feel how everything was interconnected. I could feel the Universe breathing and saw the stars dancing as we traveled through outer space. It was as if I could actually feel the Earth hurtling through space.

In these moments, some cosmic intelligence began to communicate with me. Lying there, I downloaded incredibly profound thoughts into my mind that I did not recognize as my own, but as soon as they entered my mind and I realized the profundity of them, they were gone. These thoughts and ideas were fleeting. If only I had a pen and pad on me. All I could remember was having one revelation after another, drowning in moments of "Oh my god, that's it!" only to be followed by "Wait, fuck, how did it go?!" I could do nothing but laugh at what was happening. It was like something was toying with me, reminding me that these ideas were far too great for our human minds to grasp and hold on to. I asked this intelligence to tell me everything, but it only smiled and told me my time would come, in this life or the next, but that time was not now.

As I listened and watched the stars dance, this intelligence explained that we are on a grand stage. This existence, this earthly plane, is a test of the human spirit – a place for souls to incarnate and be tested. And on this grand stage, we were being watched from above, like a mother watching her children play in the sandbox together. It look upon us with love, nothing more, nothing less. It reveled in our failures and our successes. Proud of everything we have created. This grand stage was created for souls come here to learn, and ultimately to grow. It was the greatest testament to the power of the spirit and a great reflection of the timeless duality of the light and the dark. This is a place where souls could interact with one another in the physical, in an endess web, in order to grow both individually and collectively, as it is only in the physical that many of the lessons that are necessary for the soul's ascension can take place. We carry the DNA of everyone who came before us and fight through not only our own trauma, but the trauma of all who preceded us. It is our obligation to be here, but not to be taken so seriously, because in the end that's all that this is... a test. This intelligence said to me that it could only offer love, infinitely, but the rest was up to us, as it could not control our free will. The success and failure of the human race is ultimately up to each and every one of *us*. It could only intervene in many ways, but only to guide us, not control us. I wondered if this was a higher intelligence or species communciating with me, or my higher self communicating with me. Whatever or whoever it was, the medicine had me tuned into their channel. To this day I don't know who or what it was that spoke to me, but I was a receiver of something I truly couldn't understand, and although I was loaded full of LSD, I was well aware of what was happening. Whatever "it" was smiled down on the festival – a true celebration of the human spirit. And we all smiled back.

This night changed everything for me. And The Playa, it does something to you. It filled my heart with love and acceptance for others, but more importantly, love and accetpance for myself. It reminded me that my heart is my center and that there is no greater truth than the one that sets you free. This was the moment I had been searching for all my life, without knowing it was the thing I had been searching for all my life, there, ripe for the taking, ready for me when I was ready for it, and it is always there and always will be... for all of us. We have to just be brave enough to take the plunge.

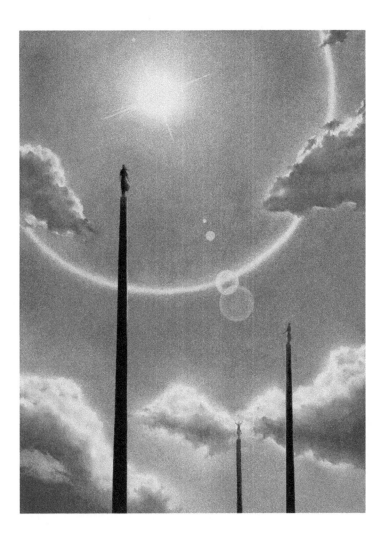

# Appendix

Appendix

# Ayahuasca
*N,N-Dimethyltryptamine*

Used as a religious sacrament for hundreds of years, Ayahuasca, known as the "vine of the souls," is a drink blend found in the Amazon made from the ayahuasca vine (*Banisteriopsis caapi*) and a shrub known as chacruna (*Psychotria viridis*). In some tribes, the ayahuasca vine is combined with chaliponga (*Diplopterys cabrerana*) to enhance and lengthen the experience. The brew is served in a ceremonial setting under the care of a shaman, also known as an ayahuasquero.

The DMT, which is the active psychedelic compound in the Ayahuasca brew, is found in the *P. viridis* shrub. When taken orally, the DMT is broken down by protective enzymes in the body; however, the *B. caapi* contains compounds that deactivate these enzymes, allowing the DMT to be orally active.

Users are recommended to follow strict preparations before a ceremony in order to improve their well-being and increase the effectiveness of the Ayahuasca brew, which includes, but is not limited to, no sexual activity, as well as no alcohol, fried foods, meat, or dairy. In some Ayahuasca brews, users experience fits of vomiting known as purging or "La Purga."

Scientific studies support the use of Ayahuasca in treating ailments such as addiction, Post-Traumatic Stress Disorder (PTSD), and depression.

*Effects can last 2-12 hours depending on potency and dosage.*

# DMT
*N,N-Dimethyltryptamine*

First synthesized by Richard Manske in 1931, DMT is a psychedelic tryptamine compound that can be found all throughout the plant and animal kingdom, as well as within humans, endogenously produced by the brain's pineal gland. What makes DMT unique is how it is actively transported across the blood-brain barrier into the brain's tissues. However, since the body contains an enzyme known as monoamine oxidase (MAO), which breaks down the DMT, the experiences are short-lived. Another form of psychedelic DMT is *5-methoxy-N,N-dimethyltryptamine*, also referred to as "5-MeO," which is an analogue of *N,N-Dimethyltryptamine* found in natural sources such as the skin and venom of the Sonoran Desert Toad.

DMT has been used ceremonially in many different cultures throughout history, such as Ayahuasca in the Amazon where it is consumed through insufflation in the form of a "snuff" or as a brew and *Acacia Nilotica* in Ancient Egypt where it is believed that Osiris, the god of rebirth, was born from an *A. Nilotica* tree. It is theorized that the burning bush in the story of Moses' divine communication with God was an acacia bush native to that region and high in DMT content. In the early 1990's, Dr. Rick Strassman led clinical trials on DMT, where patients received dosages intravenously. During these trials, detailed in the iconic book *DMT: The Spirit Molecule*, users had very similar divine visions and encounters with beings, carrying several common themes throughout their widely varying experiences.

*Effects can last 5-20 minutes depending on potency, dosage, and delivery.*

# Ibogaine
*12-Methoxyibogaine*

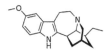

Ibogaine is a psychoactive compound found in the root bark of the Iboga shrub found in West Africa. A member of the *Apocynaceae* family, several plants contain this psychedelic compound, including *Tabernathe Iboga*, *Voacanga africana*, and *Tabernaemontana undulata*. This psychedelic compound can Used for millenia as a tribal sacrament by the members of the Bwiti religion, it is now used in today's society for the effective treatment of addiction. Although illegal in the United States as a Schedule I controlled substance, Ibogaine is legal in countries such as Canada, Mexico, Brazil, and South Africa, where many treatment centers exist.

In lower doses, studies have shown that Ibogaine has the potential to alleviate many of the physical symptoms of withdrawal and has proven to be a highly effective treatment. A study performed by MAPS found that long-term withdrawal symptoms were reduced for up to 50% of the study's participants. Studies also revealed that Ibogaine has many interactions with pharmaceuticals and has a high risk factor for people with existing cardiac conditions. In low doses, Ibogaine acts as a stimulant, but in higher doses it is a long-lasting experience, sometimes more than 24 hours, which can induce an introspective and visionary dreamlike state. It is in this state where users are able to face their internal conflicts, many of which are directly related to the addiction. Users report coming in contact with beings and being shown or taught things during these interactions.

*Effects can last up to 24 hours or more depending on potency and dosage.*

# Ketamine
*Ketamine Hydrochloride*

Ketamine, known for its hallucinogenic, dissociative, and sedative effects, is a fast-acting general anesthetic that has been used during surgery for both humans and animals. First synthesized in 1962 by Calvin Stevens, it was developed as an anesthetic and replacement to PCP.

In 1963, it was first patented in Belgium as an animal anesthetic and soon after, testing began on humans. That is when its hallucinogenic effects were discovered. While mainly used on animals, it has been used as a field anesthetic in military applications. Today, Ketamine is used on children and other adults during minor surgeries.

Studies have shown that Ketamine can be used therapeutically, effectively treating people suffering from major depression with an imminent risk of suicide. Furthermore, Ketamine has proven to work faster than other typical treatments, working within hours or days, while current anti-depressant medication can take weeks or months, although its effects may be short-lived.

Ketamine is typically taken intramuscularly, but can be consumed through other methods such as insufflation. During a non-fatal overdose, users experienced what is commonly referred to as a "K-hole," in which they experience detachment from reality and/or the body, as well as Near Death Experiences (NDEs).

*Effects can last 5-60 minutes depending on potency, dosage, and delivery.*

# LSD
*Lysergic acid diethylamide*

In 1938, while searching for a respiratory and circulatory stimulant, Swiss chemist Albert Hofmann first synthesized LSD from ergotamine, a chemical derived from a fungus found on rye and other cereals known as ergot. It was not until 1943 that he discovered its psychedelic properties. In Ancient Greece, a ritual known as the Eleusinian Mysteries took place every year for nearly two thousand years, where initiates would drink a hallucinogenic brew known as "the kykeon." The brew's recipe consisted of barley and was believed to include an ergotamine compound, which is also the main compound used to synthesize LSD. After the discovery of LSD, Hofmann pursued the notion that the psychedelic experience induced by the kykeon potion at Eleusis resulted from the same chemical makeup as that found in LSD.

In the late 1950's, Dr. Humphrey Osmond supplied LSD to members of Alcoholics Anonymous who had failed to quit drinking; through this, he discovered that LSD had a success rate of approximately 50% in treating alcoholism – an efficacy that had not been seen in any other type of treatment. LSD has been actively used in a therapeutic setting since the 1970's, and in more recent years it has been applied in the treatment of severe anxiety associated with terminal illness. Taken in low doses of 10-20 mcg, also known as "microdosing," LSD has been shown to enhance creativity, improved coordination, and increased stamina.

*Effects last from 4-12 hours depending on potency and dosage.*

# MDMA
*3,4-Methylenedioxymethamphetamine*

Widely known as "ecstasy" for its ability to induce euphoria, MDMA is a synthetic drug that acts as both a psychedelic and a stimulant, heightening the user's sense of intimacy and emotional connection with others. With a chemical structure similar to that of Methamphetamine and Mescaline, MDMA was first discovered and patented in the early 1900's by the pharmaceutical company Merck. It was found that sassafras oil can be extracted from the sassafras tree's dried root bark through the process of steam distillation in order to obtain safrole, which is the primary precursor of MDMA.

In 1965, chemist Alexander Shulgin synthesized MDMA while performing research at Dow Chemical Company, but he was not aware of its psychoactive properties. It wasn't until 1976 that Shulgin would consume MDMA and learn about its therapeutic effects, noting that it allowed the user to see the world clearly and without inhibitions. In his pursuit to find an effective therapeutic drug, Shulgin's work influenced its widespread use in Western culture. Advocates in the fields of psychology and cognitive therapy have supported the belief that MDMA holds therapeutic benefits and facilitates more effective psychotherapy sessions by comforting the user to openly discuss deeply traumatizing experiences. Clinical trials have tested the therapeutic potential of MDMA for Post-Traumatic Stress Disorder (PTSD), as well as anxiety and depression associated with terminal illness.

*Effects can last 2-6 hours depending on potency, dosage, and delivery.*

# Psilocybin

*4-phosphoryloxy-N,N-dimethyltryptamine*

Mainly found in tropical environments, there are 144 strains of hallucinogenic Psilocybin mushrooms, with over fifty found in Mexico and over fifty more found throughout Latin America and the Caribbean.

In Mesoamerica it is believed that the mushroom was used ceremonially for millennia. The Aztecs had also used a substance called Teonanácatl or "flesh of the gods" that was believed to be Psilocybin mushrooms. Archaeologists have found that the ritual use of psychedelic mushrooms is far-reaching, explicitly represented in rock paintings dating back 9,000 years in the Sahara Desert.

Psilocybin was introduced to Westerners in the 1950's by mycologist R. Gordon Wasson who had visited Mexico in search of a "magic" mushroom, ultimately observing and partaking in rituals with the local natives. His experiences were published in Life magazine in 1957 titled, "Seeking the Magic Mushroom."

In a scientific study, it was discovered that Psilocybin successfully lifted the severe depression of all of the study's participants who had been suffering from long-term depression that anti-depressant medication could not treat. Psilocybin has also been found to alleviate and cure addiction and Post-Traumatic Stress Disorder (PTSD) and is used in therapeutic settings to alleviate the fear of death in the terminally ill.

*Effects can last from 2-8 hours depending on strain, potency, dosage, and delivery.*

# Salvia
*Salvia divinorum*

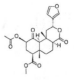

*Salvia divinorum*, also known as Sage of the Diviners, is a perennial herb indigenous to the Sierra Mazateca region of Oaxaca, Mexico. It is used ceremonially and touted for its medicinal healing properties by the Mazatec people to alleviate ailments such as anemia, cluster headaches, and diarrhea. In larger doses, Salvia can induce altered states of consciousness.

The first recorded mention of Salvia in Western culture was made by Jean Basset Johnson during his studies of Mazatec shamanism in the late 1930's where he had heard that they were drinking a brew made from a visionary tea. In 1962, Albert Hofmann and R. Gordon Wasson obtained a specimen from the Mazatecs, in which they described it as a "less desirable substitute" for Psilocybin.

Modern medicine has discovered its therapeutic properties and believes its active compounds may be used to treat opioid addiction, schizophrenia, chronic pain, and Alzheimer's disease. Salvia has also been proven to curb cravings for heroin and cocaine. Salvia, whose psychoactive component is *Salvinorin A*, can be consumed by smoking or vaporizing its dried leaves, but its effects tend to be shorter when smoked. Conversely, chewing its leaves tends to have longer lasting effects. There are significant variations in its psychoactivity based on a variety of phsyiological and consumption factors.

*Effects can last 5-120 minutes depending on potency, dosage, and delivery.*

# San Pedro

*Echinopsis pachanoi*

Known by the names *Echinopsis pachanoi* and *Trichocereus pachanoi*, San Pedro is mostly found in the Andes Mountains in South America and can grow to over six meters tall. Archaeological records indicate that San Pedro has been used in healing ceremonies by Andean cultures for over 3,000 years. Traditionally, these ceremonies are held within the presence of a shaman, known in the Peruvian Amazon as a curandero or healer, who guides the user through their experience. Indigenously known as huachuma, San Pedro can cause the user to purge, or vomit due to the effects of the plant.

The oldest depiction of the San Pedro cactus was found in a carving in the Chavin de Huantar temple in Peru and dates back to 1300 B.C. This plant received its name after a mythological tale in which God hid the keys to heaven and San Pedro (St. Peter) used the powers of the cactus to reveal the hidden location of the keys. This plant medicine was used by different cultures throughout South America not just for their spiritual psychoactive properties, but as a medicine to cure physical ailments as well.

San Pedro can be prepared by cutting slices of the cactus and boiling them in water, releasing their psychoactive compounds into a brew which can be consumed orally. It can also be consumed by drying out the cactus, where it can be ground into powder form.

*Effects can last 6-16 hours depending on the source, potency, dosage, and delivery.*

To submit your own experience to be

considered for future volumes please visit

**THE-PSYCHEDELIC-ANTHOLOGY.COM**

## Additional Resources

psymposia.com
shroomery.org
maps.org
zendoproject.org
reset.me
DMT-nexus.me
erowid.org
thethirdwave.co

CPSIA information can be obtained
at www.ICGtesting.com
Printed in the USA
FSHW010605180819
61160FS